Study Guide

to Accompany

Core Concepts in Health
Eighth Edition

Paul M. Insel and Walton T. Roth
Stanford University

prepared by
Thomas M. Davis
The University of Northern Iowa

Mayfield Publishing Company
Mountain View, California
London • Toronto

International Standard Book Number: 1-55934-907-7

Manufactured in the United States of America
10 9 8 7 6 5 4 3 2 1

Mayfield Publishing Company
1280 Villa Street
Mountain View, California 94041

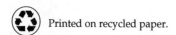 Printed on recycled paper.

CONTENTS

WELLNESS WORKSHEETS

*Worksheets that include an Internet activity

*Worksheets that include an Internet activity

*Worksheets that include an Internet activity

PREFACE

This Study Guide is designed to help you review and master the most important principles of personal health presented in *Core Concepts in Health,* Eighth Edition. The Study Guide will not only assist you in mastering the information in each chapter of the textbook but also help you use that information in your daily life.

The Study Guide is divided into two parts. The first part contains learning objectives, key terms, major points/issues, and sample test questions for each chapter:

- **Learning Objectives** indicate the main things you should know once you have read the chapter and completed the items in the Study Guide. Read through the lists of learning objectives and key terms before you begin reading each chapter. This should help you organize and pace your reading.

- The lists of **Key Terms** should help you in your reading of the chapter and in studying for exams. You may find it helpful to jot down brief definitions (or page numbers where definitions appear) as you read through the chapter.

- The lists of **Major Points/Issues** can help you review the key topics discussed in each chapter. If you find any of the listed points unfamiliar or confusing, reread the appropriate portions of the textbook chapter.

- The **Sample Test Questions** can serve both as a review of chapter content and as practice for examinations. An answer key is provided to allow you to check your answers. The sample test questions can help show you what areas of each chapter you need to review further. To help you with that review, each answer in the answer key has a textbook page number reference to guide you in finding information relevant to answering that question.

The second part of the Study Guide contains ninety Wellness Worksheets. Most of the worksheets provide additional assessment tools to help you learn more about your health-related attitudes and behaviors. Others are strictly knowledge-based and will help you test your comprehension of key concepts. Selected worksheets include Internet activities that you can use to find wellness-related information on the World Wide Web. By completing the worksheets, you will gain a better grasp of important concepts and will be better prepared to implement a successful behavior change program.

Chapter 1
Taking Charge of Your Health

LEARNING OBJECTIVES

As a result of reading Chapter 1 in the textbook and completing the activities in this Study Guide, you should be able to do the following:

1. Compare and contrast today's ideas about wellness with those held about health a century ago.

2. Provide supporting evidence for the belief that the best treatment for degenerative diseases (the major cause of death and disability today) is living a healthy lifestyle.

3. Define the concept known as *wellness,* and describe its six dimensions.

4. Describe the primary habits and behaviors of a wellness lifestyle.

5. Discuss the multidimensional nature of wellness, and provide examples of healthful behaviors for each dimension.

6. Identify the major goals of the national *Healthy People 2000* program.

7. Describe the interrelationships among behavioral, hereditary, and environmental factors for a given health problem.

8. List the rewards associated with a wellness lifestyle.

9. Explain the importance of personal decision making and behavior change in achieving a wellness lifestyle.

10. Discuss the significance of motivation and commitment in the process of behavior change.

11. Describe Prochaska's Stages of Change model.

12. Create a behavior management plan to change a health behavior.

13. Name at least five strategies you can use to increase your chances of successful behavior change.

14. Describe the influence that factors such as gender, socioeconomic status, ethnicity, and age have on health.

15. Describe the actions you can take, as an individual, to help create a more healthful environment.

TERMINOLOGY

You should be able to define the following key terms:

action stage
commitment
contemplation stage
emotional wellness
environmental or planetary wellness
intellectual wellness
interpersonal and social wellness
locus of control
maintenance stage

motivation
personal wellness contract
physical wellness
precontemplation stage
preparation stge
spiritual wellness
target behavior
termination stage
wellness

MAJOR POINTS/ISSUES

1. Wellness is multidimensional; wellness is more than physical fitness.

2. The national health objectives published in *Healthy People 2000* set measurable standards for facilitating the best possible health for Americans.

3. A variety of factors influence our health, including environment, heredity, and access to health care, but the most significant determinant of our health is our behavior.

4. Changing behavior doesn't happen by luck. People can plan for behavior change, and Prochaska's Stages of Change model is one way to understand and plan for successful behavior change.

5. People with an internal locus of control make decisions to serve their own best interests. People with an external locus of control respond to outside forces in making decisions, sometimes not in their own best interests.

6. Motivation and commitment are important factors in behavior change.

7. Positive health behaviors can be initiated and successfully maintained through a systematic program of behavior self-management. There are six basic steps in a behavior change program: (1) monitor behavior and gather data, (2) analyze the data and identify patterns, (3) set specific goals, (4) devise a plan of action, (5) modify your environment, and (6) involve people around you.

8. Chances for successful behavior change can be increased by focusing on one target behavior, controlling environmental stimuli, setting up rewards, using a buddy system and a role model, and expecting success.

9. Common obstacles for change include nonsupportive people, low level of commitment, inappropriate techniques, stress, procrastination, rationalizing, and blaming.

10. Some behaviors are too deeply rooted to be changed by self-management techniques alone and may require getting outside help.

11. Starting and maintaining a behavior change program requires commitment, a well-developed plan, social support, and a system of rewards.

SAMPLE TEST QUESTIONS

Completion

1. An outdated definition of health describes it as an absence of _____ disease.

2. Improving and balancing the intellectual, physical, emotional, interpersonal, environmental, and spiritual dimensions of your life is to fulfill your potential for _____.

3. Choosing a nutritious diet, preventing injuries to one's self, and getting regular medical checkups are examples of _____ wellness.

4. Having a sense of humor, creativity, and curiosity are characteristics of _____ wellness.

5. Possessing effective communication skills and having a capacity for intimacy are characteristic of _____ wellness.

6. Increasing the healthy life span of Americans, reducing health disparities, and securing access to preventive health services are the major goals outlined in a federal document titled: _____.

7. If a person believes that suffering a serious illness is just a matter of luck, he or she might be characterized as having an _____ locus of control.

8. From the early 1970s until 1993, the death rate in America fell primarily due to _____.

9. The leading cause of death in the United States is _____.

10. Factors other than behavior that affect wellness are heredity, access to adequate health care, and _____.

True or False

1. Intellectual wellness and emotional wellness are essentially the same thing.

2. The concept of wellness is relatively new.

3. Increasing every Americans' access to expensive, life-extending medical treatments is one of the national health objectives.

4. Possessing a personal wellness profile is defined primarily by a high level of cardiovascular fitness.

5. The first stage of Prochaska's Stages of Change model is precontemplation.

6. Internal locus of control might be described as a high level of perceived personal control of events that happen in a person's life.

7. Personal health contracts tend to set people up for failure by creating expectations that cannot be fulfilled.

8. Some health behaviors are difficult or impossible to change without outside assistance.

9. A single person's influence over planetary wellness is so insignificant that it doesn't really matter what individual choices people make related to the environment.

10. In the mid-1990s the death rate rose for several reasons including the epidemic of HIV infections and subsequent AIDS diagnoses.

Multiple Choice

1. All of the following are dimensions of wellness described in the book EXCEPT:
   a. planetary wellness
   b. emotional wellness
   c. interpersonal wellness
   d. socioeconomic wellness

2. Self-acceptance is MOST representative of:
   a. physical wellness
   b. emotional wellness
   c. intellectual wellness
   d. spiritual wellness

3. Which of the following is NOT one of the primary broad goals of *Healthy People 2000?*
   a. increasing access to preventive health care
   b. increasing the span of healthy life of all Americans
   c. increasing health insurance options for all Americans
   d. decreasing health disparities among Americans

4. The MOST important contributor to the wellness of most people is:
   a. health behavior
   b. health care
   c. heredity
   d. environment

5. In Prochaska's Stages of Change model, people who are denying the problem exists are in the _____ stage.
   a. precontemplation
   b. contemplation
   c. preparation
   d. action

6. Which of the following is an example of internal locus of control? Believing that:
   a. There is really nothing I can do to avoid getting cancer.
   b. Some power greater than self will decide when a person will die.
   c. Smoking behaviors can be attributed to advertising.
   d. Healthy living can prevent colds.

7. A target behavior may best be described as:
   a. the risky behavior of a loved one that you would like to see changed
   b. your own risky behavior you would like to change
   c. the thing you do that is most risky
   d. a risky behavior that your family or employer tries to get you to change

8. Stress barriers:
   a. should be anticipated and should not slow your progress in changing behavior
   b. may temporarily prevent you from reaching a short-term goal
   c. are mental pressures that can best be handled through ignoring them
   d. affect everyone the same way

9. An out-of-date definition of health is:
   a. fulfillment of personal potential
   b. personal wellness
   c. being without symptoms
   d. multidimensional

10. The steps on the wellness continuum between "average" and "high level of wellness" are:
    a. change and growth; vital meaningful life
    b. change and growth; physical and mental symptoms
    c. vital meaningful life; malaise
    d. physical and mental symptoms; malaise

SAMPLE TEST QUESTIONS ANSWER KEY

Completion

1. physical (p. 2)
2. wellness (pp. 2–3)
3. physical (p. 2)
4. intellectual (p. 2)
5. interpersonal (p. 3)
6. *Healthy People 2000: National Health Promotion and Disease Prevention Objectives* (pp. 5–7)
7. external (p. 11)
8. healthier lifestyles (p. 4)
9. heart disease (p. 7)
10. environment (p. 6)

True or False

1. F (p. 2)
2. T (p. 3)
3. F (pp. 5–7)
4. F (pp. 9–10)
5. T (p. 10)
6. T (p. 12)
7. F (p. 16)
8. T (p. 19)
9. F (p. 20)
10. T (p. 4)

Multiple Choice

1. d (pp. 2–3)
2. b (p. 2)
3. c (pp. 5–6)
4. a (p. 6)
5. a (p. 10)
6. d (p. 12)
7. b (p. 13)
8. b (p. 18)
9. c (p. 4)
10. a (p. 2)

Turn to the back of the Study Guide, and complete Wellness Worksheets 1–6.

Chapter 2
Stress: The Constant Challenge

LEARNING OBJECTIVES

As a result of reading Chapter 2 in the textbook and completing the activities in this Study Guide, you should be able to do the following:

1. Describe stress.

2. Describe how people react to stress physically, emotionally, and behaviorally.

3. Describe the relationship between stress and disease.

4. Describe the relationship between personality types and stress in one's life.

5. Identify common sources of stress.

6. Describe techniques for preventing and managing stress.

7. Prepare a step-by-step plan for successfully managing the stress in your life.

TERMINOLOGY

You should be able to define the following key terms:

adrenal glands
adrenocorticotropic hormone (ACTH)
alarm
atherosclerosis
autonomic nervous system
biofeedback
burnout
cortisol
desensitization
distress
endocrine system
endorphins
epinephrine
eustress
exhaustion
fight-or-flight reaction
gender role
general adaptation syndrome
hardy personality

homeostasis
hormone
hypothalamus
meditation
mind-body connection
norepinephrine
parasympathetic division
pituitary gland
psychoneuroimmunology
relaxation response
repetitive-strain injury (RSI)
resistance
somatic nervous system
stress
stress response
stressor
sympathetic division
Type A and Type B personalities
visualization

MAJOR POINTS/ISSUES

1. Stressful situations can be psychological or physical and may be perceived as pleasant as well as unpleasant.

2. We inherently respond to stressful situations with a fight-or-flight reaction, even though such a response is often not appropriate in contemporary society.

3. The body attempts to maintain homeostasis; stress is an internal or external disruption in the body's steady state.

4. How people respond to stressful circumstances varies widely depending on many factors including the severity of the stressor, one's perception of the stressor, personality, cultural background, and past experiences with similar or other stressors.

5. The General Adaptation Syndrome is one model for describing how organisms respond to stress. The states of the General Adaptation Syndrome are alarm, resistance, and exhaustion.

6. Psychoneuroimmunology is the theory that stress impairs the body's immune system, increasing a person's susceptibility to disease.

7. Stress contributes to the risk of suffering from several diseases, including cardiovascular disease, colds, asthma, allergies, and some forms of cancer.

8. Stressors are common in day-to-day life and occur with great frequency in the lives of most college students.

9. The effects of stress may be reduced through the effective use of social support, good communication skills, exercise, good nutrition, getting enough sleep, and effective time management.

10. Relaxation techniques are effective in reducing the negative impact of stress. They include meditation, deep breathing, biofeedback, autogenic training, massage, music therapy, and hypnosis.

SAMPLE TEST QUESTIONS

Completion

1. A situation that triggers a physical and/or emotional reaction is called a

   _____, and the reaction itself is called the _____.

2. The branch of the autonomic nervous system that triggers the stress response is the

   _____.

3. If the body's systems are calm, with heart rate, respiration, blood pressure, and hormone levels at a normal level, the body may be described as being in _____.

4. In the face of stress, the body prepares itself to do battle or to escape the stress. This response is called the _____ reaction.

5. A person who is competitive, impatient, and sometimes hostile is a _____ personality.

6. People who believe that events in their lives are controlled primarily by forces beyond their personal control are said to have an _____ locus of control.

7. The stress of managing a huge financial inheritance is called _____.

8. The theory that stress increases susceptibility to disease by impairing the immune system is called _____.

9. A stress-management technique similar to day dreaming is _____.

10. Measurement of mostly involuntary bodily responses such as heart rate, blood pressure, and muscular tension is part of this relaxation technique: _____.

True or False

1. The parasympathetic division of the autonomic nervous system is that portion that triggers the fight-or-flight reaction.

2. A high level of stress strengthens the immune system, preventing colds and other infections.

3. People with hardy personalities are less likely to have an external locus of control.

4. According to *Healthy People 2000,* about 10% of Americans suffer adverse health effects due to stress every year.

5. Eustress is negative stress.

6. Type A personalities, with an angry and/or hostile component to that personality type, are more likely to suffer heart attacks.

7. Chronic stress puts people at elevated risk for a wide variety of negative health conditions including hives and cancer.

8. Progressive relaxation is a technique that starts relaxation with the body, specifically muscles, as a means of relaxing the mind.

9. Biofeedback measures the body's mostly involuntary functions, such as heart rate and respiration.

10. During the stress response, saliva and mucus production are reduced.

Multiple Choice

1. Our behavioral responses are managed by our:
   a. autonomic nervous system
   b. parasympathetic division
   c. sympathetic division
   d. somatic nervous system

2. The portion of our nervous system that triggers the stress response is the
   _____.
   a. autonomic nervous system
   b. parasympathetic division
   c. sympathetic division
   d. somatic nervous system

3. Which of the following characteristics is MOST closely associated with the Type A personality?
   a. tolerance
   b. optimism
   c. sense of inner purpose
   d. cynicism

4. Repetitive-strain injury (RSI) is MOST likely to affect the sense of:
   a. hearing
   b. sight
   c. touch
   d. smell

5. Which of the following is one of the stages of the General Adaptation Syndrome?
   a. anxiety
   b. ambivalence
   c. stabilization
   d. alarm

6. Eustress might be triggered by:
   a. getting a bad grade
   b. winning the lottery
   c. having your parents get a divorce
   d. experiencing homeostasis

7. The stress responses produce:
   a. bronchial constriction
   b. skeletal muscle relaxation
   c. increased digestion
   d. increased respiration

8. The biggest time-management problem for most people is:
   a. scheduling
   b. too many things to do
   c. procrastination
   d. conflicting values

9. Another term for imagery is:
   a. progressive relaxation
   b. visualization
   c. meditation
   d. biofeedback

10. Which of the following is NOT a health condition linked to stress?
    a. asthma
    b. digestive problems
    c. headaches
    d. changes in vision

SAMPLE TEST QUESTIONS ANSWER KEY

Completion

1. stressor, stress response (p. 26)
2. sympathetic division (p. 27)
3. homeostasis (p. 28)
4. fight-or-flight (p. 29)
5. Type A (p. 30)
6. external (p. 30)
7. eustress (p. 32)
8. psychoneuroimmunology (p. 32)
9. visualization (pp. 43–44)
10. biofeedback (p. 45)

True or False

1. F (p. 27)
2. F (pp. 32–33)
3. T (p. 30)
4. F (p. 32)
5. F (p. 32)
6. T (p. 34)
7. T (pp. 33–35)
8. T (p. 43)
9. T (p. 45)
10. T (p. 28)

Multiple Choice

1. a (p. 29)
2. c (p. 27)
3. d (p. 30)
4. c (p. 34)
5. d (p. 32)
6. a (p. 32)
7. d (p. 28)
8. c (p. 41)
9. b (pp. 43–44)
10. d (pp. 34–35)

Turn to the back of the Study Guide, and complete Wellness Worksheets 7–12.

Chapter 3
Psychological Health

LEARNING OBJECTIVES

As a result of reading Chapter 3 in the textbook and completing the activities in this Study Guide, you should be able to do the following:

1. Describe what it means to be psychologically healthy.

2. Explain how to develop and maintain a positive self-concept and high self-esteem.

3. Discuss the importance to psychological health of an optimistic outlook, good communication skills, and constructive approaches to dealing with anger.

4. Describe common psychological disorders, and list danger signals of suicide.

5. Explain different models of human nature and how they influence approaches to therapy for psychological problems.

6. Describe the different types of help available for psychological problems.

TERMINOLOGY

You should be able to define the following key terms:

anxiety	mania
assertiveness	normality
auditory hallucinations	obsession
authenticity	obsessive-compulsive disorder
autonomy	other-directed
behavioral model	panic disorder
bipolar disorder	phobia
biological model	post-traumatic stress disorder
cognitive distortion	psychological health
cognitive model	psychoanalytic model
compulsion	reinforcement
creativity	response
defense mechanism	schizophrenia
delusions	self-actualization
depression	self-concept
desensitization	self-esteem
deteriorating social and work functioning	self-talk
exposure	stimulus
inner-directed	unconscious

MAJOR POINTS/ISSUES

1. Psychological health encompasses more than normality. Psychological diversity is valuable; conformity is not necessarily admirable.

2. Just as physical health is more than the absence of physical illness, psychological health is more than the absence of mental illness.

3. Maslow's hierarchy of needs, with self-actualization being the highest level, provides a good basis for definition of mental health.

4. Erik Erikson proposed that human development proceeds through eight stages, extending throughout the life span. Successful resolution of the early stages is important as the basis for successful resolution of subsequent stages.

5. Positive self-esteem, essential for good psychological health, develops during childhood as a result of giving and receiving love and learning to accomplish goals.

6. Defense mechanisms can be useful in temporarily coping but should not be allowed to prevent us from finding long-lasting solutions to challenging situations.

7. Dealing with your own anger effectively means finding a balance between suppressing your feelings out of concern for offending others and lashing out indiscriminately without regard for the rights of others.

8. People are affected by a variety of psychological disorders including schizophrenia, phobias, panic disorder, obsessions, post-traumatic stress disorder, and depression.

9. Suicide is a serious potential consequence of depression and may be indicated by expressions about suicide, social isolation, previous suicide attempts, previous suicide of a friend or relative, access to a means of killing one's self, drug or alcohol addiction, or an unexplainable improvement in one's mood.

10. Theorists have proposed four models of human nature (biological, behavioral, cognitive, and psychoanalytic) to describe psychological health and mental illness. Each model represents certain truths about human behavior. The most appropriate therapy depends on the situation.

11. Some psychological health problems can be resolved through self-help efforts, including support groups, reading self-help books, and communicating with friends, relatives, or others who have had similar experiences, including peer counseling relationships.

12. Seeking professional help for a mental or emotional problem is a matter of individual choice and, although often difficult to initiate, may be a sign of wellness.

13. Strong indications that professional help may be needed include the following: the problem interferes with daily activities, suicide has been attempted or seriously considered, symptoms such as hallucinations, delusions, incoherent speech, or loss of memory occur, and/or use of drugs is involved.

14. Mental health professionals have various forms of training; it takes time to choose an appropriate therapist, and changing therapists is sometimes necessary.

SAMPLE TEST QUESTIONS

Completion

1. According to Maslow, the full realization of one's potential is called
   _____.

2. In Maslow's hierarchy of needs, the most urgent need is _____.

3. A criterion of good psychological health is autonomy. Such people are said to be
   _____-directed.

4. Avoidance, sublimation, and humor are examples of _____ mechanisms.

5. Extreme fear of public speaking is an example of a/an _____ phobia.

6. People who suffer from panic disorders usually first experience them in the
   _____ decade of life.

7. The combination of depression, a drug addiction history, and a recent, unexplained lightening of mood may indicate a person is contemplating _____.

8. Swinging between mania and depression is a _____ disorder.

9. Of the four popular models of human behavior, the _____ model emphasizes that the mind's activity depends on the brain, the composition of which is dependent on genes.

10. Of the four popular models of human behavior, the use of reinforcement is most closely related to the _____ model.

True or False

1. Normality is a criterion for determining psychological health.

2. Self-acceptance is a prerequisite for positive psychological health.

3. Maslow's most important contribution to the study of psychological health is the description of an eight-stage model for tracking human development.

4. Erikson's life stages ended with the establishment of human identity.

5. "I won the speech contest because none of the other speakers was very good" is an example of negative self-talk.

6. Assertiveness and aggressiveness are the same thing.

7. Psychologically healthy people are able to suppress their anger to prevent hurting other's feelings.

8. Manic behavior is characterized by lethargy.

9. Schizophrenia is most frequently demonstrated by a "split personality."

10. Of the four popular models of human behavior described in the text, the least currently accepted is the psychoanalytic model.

Multiple Choice

1. All of the following are models of human nature discussed in the textbook EXCEPT:
   a. evolutionary
   b. cognitive
   c. behavioral
   d. biological

2. Which of the following is the LEAST closely associated with the behavioral model?
   a. analysis
   b. stimulus
   c. response
   d. reinforcement

3. Which of the following may be symptomatic of depression?
   a. poor appetite
   b. weight loss
   c. loss of sexual drive
   d. all of the above

4. The scientist/author associated with self-actualization is:
   a. Maslow
   b. Skinner
   c. McCluan
   d. Toffler

5. The MOST urgent need on Maslow's hierarchy of needs is:
   a. physiological needs
   b. safety
   c. being loved
   d. maintaining self-esteem

6. Self-actualized people are:
   a. critical
   b. verbal
   c. realistic
   d. self-absorbed

7. A phobia is:
   a. an unfounded fear of a specific thing
   b. a heart attack symptom
   c. a common response to stress
   d. uncommon among panic patients

8. Achieving healthy self-esteem involves all of the following EXCEPT:
   a. developing a positive self-concept
   b. meeting challenges to self-esteem
   c. developing defense mechanisms
   d. learning to deal with anger

9. An example of negative self-talk is:
   a. I overdid it last night. Next time I'll make different choices.
   b. It may not be the best speech I'll ever give, but it was good enough to earn a grade of "A."
   c. I wonder why my boss wants to see me? I'll just have to wait and see.
   d. I wouldn't feel so lousy today if someone had stopped me from drinking so much last night.

10. Which of the following describes a treatment for fear that involves coming into direct contact with the fear-inducing element?
    a. desensitization
    b. exposure
    c. self-actualization
    d. reinforcement

SAMPLE TEST QUESTIONS ANSWER KEY

Completion

1. self-actualization (p. 54)
2. physiological (p. 54)
3. inner (p. 56)
4. defense (p. 60)
5. social (p. 64)
6. third (p. 64)
7. suicide (p. 66)
8. bipolar (p. 68)
9. biological (pp. 69–70)
10. behavioral (p. 71)

True or False

1. F (p. 54)
2. T (p. 55)
3. F (p. 54)
4. F (pp. 56–57)
5. T (p. 61)
6. F (p. 63)
7. F (pp. 63–64)
8. F (p. 68)
9. F (p. 69)
10. T (p. 72)

Multiple Choice

1. a (pp. 69–72)
2. a (p. 71)
3. d (p. 66)
4. a (p. 54)
5. a (p.54)
6. c (p. 54)
7. a (p. 64)
8. c (pp. 58–60)
9. d (p. 61)
10. b (p. 71)

Turn to the back of the Study Guide, and complete Wellness Worksheets 13–19.

Chapter 4
Intimate Relationships

LEARNING OBJECTIVES

As a result of reading Chapter 4 in the textbook and completing the activities in this Study Guide, you should be able to do the following:

1. Explain the qualities that help people develop intimate relationships.

2. Discuss the relationship between self-image, self-esteem, and the success of personal relationships.

3. Identify the predictors of successful friendships.

4. Describe different types of love relationships and the stages they often go through.

5. Identify the roots of jealousy and describe the potential effect of jealousy on a relationship.

6. Identify the characteristics that people usually seek in intimate partners.

7. Describe the changing acceptance of cohabitation, including the kinds of people who are most likely to cohabit.

8. Describe the similarities between heterosexual and homosexual relationships.

9. Discuss relationship options available to adults today.

10. Describe the criteria of a successful marriage.

11. Identify the special challenges of single parenting.

12. List some characteristics of successful families as well as some potential problems families face.

TERMINOLOGY

You should be able to define the following key terms:

affiliative conversation	fatuous
attachment	gay
cohabitation	gender role
commitment	heterosexual
diversity	homosexual
divorce	infatuation

intimacy
jealousy
lesbian
love transformation
nonmarital partnerships
reciprocity

self-esteem
self-image
separation
sexual orientation
singlehood

MAJOR POINTS/ISSUES

1. Intimate relationships are important to people's relationships and well-being.

2. Self-image and self-esteem are important prerequisites to the development of successful relationships.

3. Friendships are based on common interests, mutual acceptance, and feelings of respect and satisfaction.

4. Love includes intimacy, trust, caring, respect, and loyalty.

5. Intense love is usually accompanied by physiological arousal. Familiarity gradually diminishes excitement.

6. Love relationships change over time, with passion decreasing and intimacy increasing. Commitment may increase or decrease.

7. Partners are likely to have more similarities than differences.

8. Cohabitation is increasing among people of all ages, with a variety of factors motivating people to live together without getting married.

9. Long-term gay and lesbian relationships are more like heterosexual relationships than different.

10. People perceive singlehood to have a variety of advantages, including freedom in decision making and freedom to have a variety of sexual partners.

11. Love is not enough to ensure success in marriage, but marriage can provide affection, affirmation, sexual fulfillment, and the opportunity for childbearing.

12. Communication skills are essential to successful relationships, and keys to communication include self-disclosure, listening, and feedback.

13. Conflict is inevitable in relationships. Conflict-resolution skills are important in maintaining relationships.

14. Families are of many styles, including traditional, blended or stepfamilies, and single-parent families.

15. Important qualities in successful families include commitment, appreciation, communication, time spent together, spiritual wellness, and skills in dealing with stress and crisis.

SAMPLE TEST QUESTIONS

Completion

1. A positive self-concept and high _____ help us to respect and love others.

2. The activities and characteristics our culture deems appropriate for us, based on whether we're male or female is called our _____.

3. Sternberg has proposed that love is composed of _____, _____, and _____.

4. The most comprehensive form of love, according to Sternberg, is _____ love.

5. When our verbal and nonverbal messages are incongruent, our messages are said to be _____.

6. Living together before marriage is called _____.

7. The second greatest stressor in life, after death of a spouse, is _____.

8. The family members for whom divorce is most traumatic are the _____.

9. Single parenthood is usually a _____ stage. The majority of male and female single parents remarry.

10. Marital satisfaction for couples with children is most likely to decline when children reach _____ age.

True or False

1. One's gender role is defined by one's feelings

2. According to Sternberg, fatuous and companionate love are the same.

3. Passion, intimacy, and commitment follow parallel paths in their intensity through the life of a relationship.

4. People with high self-esteem are less likely to feel jealous.

5. The majority of our communication may be nonverbal.

6. A first step in conflict resolution is clarifying issues.

7. Cohabitating couples who plan to marry feel less satisfaction than married couples.

8. The emotional nature of homosexual relationships is like that of heterosexual relationships.

9. The largest share of single adult Americans have never been married.

10. About 30% of all people who divorce eventually remarry.

Multiple Choice

1. Our gender role is defined for us by our:
   a. genetics
   b. culture
   c. decisions
   d. sexual experiences

2. Which of the following is NOT one of Sternberg's three elements of love?
   a. passion
   b. intimacy
   c. commitment
   d. communication

3. Which of the following is probably LEAST important in maintaining good communication in a relationship?
   a. desensitization
   b. self-disclosure
   c. listening skills
   d. feedback

4. One of the first elements to begin to cause attraction between two people is:
   a. social status
   b. political persuasion
   c. personality traits
   d. general behavior

5. The factor that MOST separates people who cohabit from those who don't is:
   a. age
   b. sexual orientation
   c. religiousness
   d. gender

6. The adoption of "best friends" roles in a relationship is MOST often found in:
   a. long-term marriages
   b. cohabitating couples
   c. relationships that have just begun
   d. gay and lesbian relationships

7. MOST families are:
   a. intact
   b. single-parent households
   c. stepfamilies
   d. gay couples

8. Marital satisfaction is likely to be at its lowest:
   a. before children are born
   b. when children are babies
   c. when children are school age
   d. after children are adults

9. Regarding families, which of the following statements is MOST true?
   a. Financial challenges are the biggest problems for both single parent fathers and mothers.
   b. Children with two parents in the household are better off regardless of the quality of the relationship with their parents.
   c. Stepfamilies are significantly different from intact families.
   d. There are no real predictors of which families will be successful.

10. People who live alone or who do not enjoy the support of others are more likely to die from:
    a. heart attacks
    b. smoking-related cancers
    c. breast cancer
    d. all of the above

SAMPLE TEST QUESTIONS ANSWER KEY

Completion

1. self-esteem (p. 82)
2. gender role (p. 82)
3. intimacy, passion, commitment (p. 84)
4. consummate (p. 84)
5. mixed (p. 87)
6. cohabitation (p. 90)
7. divorce (p. 94)
8. children (p. 95)
9. transitional (p. 97)
10. school (p. 96)

True or False

1. F (p. 82)
2. F (p. 84)
3. F (p. 84)
4. T (p. 86)
5. T (p. 86)
6. T (p. 88)
7. F (p. 92)
8. T (p. 92)
9. T (p. 92)
10. F (p. 95)

Multiple Choice

1. b (p. 82)
2. d (p. 84)
3. a (p. 87)
4. a (p. 89)
5. c (p. 90)
6. d (p. 92)
7. a (p. 95)
8. c (p. 96)
9. c (p. 97)
10. d (p. 94)

Turn to the back of the Study Guide, and complete Wellness Worksheets 20–24.

Chapter 5
Sex and Your Body

LEARNING OBJECTIVES

As a result of reading Chapter 5 in the textbook and completing the activities in this Study Guide, you should be able to do the following:

1. Describe the structure and function of the female and male sexual organs.

2. Describe the influence of hormones on sexual responsiveness.

3. Describe the process of sexual development.

4. Explain the changes in sexual functioning that occur across the life span.

5. Describe how the sex organs function during sexual activity and list the common causes of sexual problems.

6. Outline the factors that influence sexual behavior and the various ways human sexuality can be expressed.

7. Describe guidelines for safe, responsible sexual behavior.

TERMINOLOGY

You should be able to define the following key terms:

adrenal glands
anal intercourse
androgens
androgyny
atypical sexual behavior
autoeroticism
bisexual
Candida
celibacy
cervix
chlamydia
chromosomes
circumcision
clitoris
corpus luteum
Cowper's glands
cunnilingus
dysmenorrhea
endocrine glands

endometriosis
epididymis
erectile dysfunction
erogenous zone
erotic fantasy
estrogens
excitement phase
fallopian tubes
fellatio
female circumcision
follicle-stimulating hormone (FSH)
foreplay
foreskin
Gardnerella
gay liberation
gender
gender identity
gender role
germ cells

glans
gonadotropic hormones
gonadotropin-releasing hormone (GnRH)
gonads
heterosexual
homophobia
homosexual
hormones
human chorionic gonadotropin (HCG)
hymen
hypothalamus
infertility
labia majora
labia minora
luteinizing hormone (LH)
masturbation
menarche
menopause
menses
menstrual cycle
menstruation
mons pubis
myotonia
nocturnal emissions
oral-genital stimulation
orgasm
orgasmic dysfunction
orgasmic phase
osteoporosis
ova
ovary
oviduct
ovulation
paraphilia
pelvic inflammatory disease (PID)
penis
pheromones
physical stimulation
pituitary gland
plateau phase
pornography
preejaculatory fluid

premature ejaculation
premenstrual syndrome (PMS)
premenstrual tension
prepuce
progesterone
progestins
prostate gland
prostatitis
prostitution
psychological stimulation
puberty
rape
refractory period
resolution phase
retarded ejaculation
scrotum
semen
seminal vesicles
sex
sex chromosomes
sex hormones
sexual anatomy
sexual arousal
sexual coercion
sexual disorder
sexual dysfunction
sexual intercourse
sexual orientation
sexuality
sperm
testis
testicular cancer
testosterone
urethra (female)
urethra (male)
uterus
vagina
vaginismus
vaginitis
vas deferens
vasocongestion
vulva

MAJOR POINTS/ISSUES

1. Sexuality plays a basic role in human life from conception to death.

2. Knowledge about the body's sexual functioning is vital to a healthy life.

3. Sexuality is a complex configuration of inborn, biological characteristics and acquired behaviors that are learned in the course of growing up in a particular family, community, and society.

4. The sexual organs of males and females develop from the same structures and fulfill similar functions.

5. Sexual functions are integrated parts of the whole body's operations.

6. In response to effective physical and/or psychological stimulation, the body shows a predictable set of sexual responses.

7. Sex hormones greatly influence the development and function of the reproductive system.

8. Sex differentiation is a process that begins at conception and proceeds, under the direction of hormones, through puberty.

9. Aging has predictable effects on human sexuality for both men and women, although it need not signal an end to sexual pleasure.

10. The role of hormones in sexual behavior is complicated by the enormous influence of cultural learning on behavior.

11. Both physical and psychological problems can interfere with sexual functioning.

12. Most forms of sexual disorders and dysfunctions can be successfully treated.

13. Sexual competence is learned; new patterns of sexual behavior can be learned through sex therapy.

14. Sexual interaction occurs in heterosexual, homosexual, and bisexual patterns. Homosexuals, as well as heterosexuals, often develop long-term relationships with one other person.

15. Many different theories attempt to account for the development of sexual orientation, but a definitive answer has yet to be provided.

16. Responsible sexual behavior includes honest communication, commonly agreed-upon sexual activities, contraception and safer sex practices, and taking responsibility for the consequences of your sexual behavior.

SAMPLE TEST QUESTIONS

Completion

1. The female gonads are called the _____.

2. All human cells ordinarily contain 23 pairs of _____.

3. The four phases of the menstrual cycle include menses, estrogenic, ovulation, and _____.

4. Male sexual maturation usually begins about _____ years after female.

5. The end of menstruation in the life of a female is called _____.

6. The four phases of the sexual response cycle include the excitement, plateau, orgasmic, and _____ phases.

7. The contemporary term for impotence is _____ dysfunction.

8. Your personal, inner sense of your gender role is your gender _____.

9. People who are sexually attracted to both sexes are _____.

10. Stimulation of the female genitals with the lips and tongue is called

_____.

True or False

1. The function of the scrotum is to keep the testes at a lower temperature than the rest of the body.

2. The majority of the world's male babies are not circumcised.

3. The sex of a person is determined at conception.

4. Males begin to mature sexually at approximately the same age as females.

5. Research into the cause of PMS has focused on hormonal, nutritional, and psychological factors.

6. The orgasmic phase is the last phase of the sexual response cycle.

7. Women do not experience a refractory period after an orgasm.

8. Gender role and gender identity are the same thing.

9. Homosexual experiences in early adolescence is a clear indication that the person will always prefer same-sex encounters.

10. Recent research has proven that sexual orientation is determined solely by genetic factors.

Multiple Choice

1. Day one of the menstrual cycle occurs during the _____.
   a. menses
   b. estrogenic phase
   c. ovulation phase
   d. progestational phase

2. The cause of PMS is:
   a. hormonal fluctuations
   b. life stress
   c. heavy menstrual bleeding
   d. unknown

3. The phase of the sexual cycle unique to men is:
   a. resolution
   b. plateau
   c. refractory
   d. excitement

4. Vaginitis may be caused by:
   a. *Candida*
   b. *Trichomonas*
   c. *Gardnerella*
   d. all of the above

5. The primary difference between homosexuals and heterosexuals is:
   a. intellectual
   b. appearance
   c. erotic partner choice
   d. values

6. The percent of college students who masturbate several times a week is approximately _____.
   a. 12%
   b. 25%
   c. 53%
   d. 67%

7. Adolescent sexual behavior:
   a. includes intercourse for less than 25% of adolescents
   b. is influenced by factors such as peer pressure
   c. is a reliable predictor of adult sexual orientation
   d. includes masturbation among boys but not girls

8. Prostitutes may be:
   a. men
   b. women
   c. children
   d. all of the above

9. The first sign of puberty in females is:
   a. breast development
   b. menstruation
   c. hair growth
   d. body growth

10. Data indicate that the sexual motives of love and physical gratification are approximately equal in males and females in the _____ age range.
    a. 21–25
    b. 26–30
    c. 31–35
    d. 36–40

SAMPLE TEST QUESTIONS ANSWER KEY

Completion

1. ovaries (p. 104)
2. chromosomes (p. 107)
3. progestational (p. 108)
4. two (p. 110)
5. menopause (p. 111)
6. resolution (p. 114)
7. erectile (p. 115)
8. identity (p. 116)
9. bisexual (p. 121)
10. cunnilingus (p. 123)

True or False

1. T (p. 105)
2. T (p. 107)
3. T (p. 108)
4. F (p. 110)
5. T (p. 110)
6. F (p. 114)
7. T (p. 114)
8. F (p. 116)
9. F (p. 119)
10. F (p. 122)

Multiple Choice

1. a (p. 108)
2. d (p. 110)
3. c (p. 114)
4. d (p. 114)
5. c (p. 121)
6. d (p. 123)
7. b (p. 119)
8. d (p. 125)
9. a (p. 108)
10. d (p. 120)

Turn to the back of the Study Guide, and complete Wellness Worksheets 25–27.

Chapter 6
Contraception

LEARNING OBJECTIVES

As a result of reading Chapter 6 in the textbook and completing the activities in this Study Guide, you should be able to do the following:

1. Explain the basic principle underlying each of the four approaches to contraception: barrier methods, hormonal methods, surgical methods, and natural methods.

2. Discuss the important issues to be considered when choosing a contraceptive.

3. Describe the advantages and disadvantages of the following types of contraception:
    a. oral contraceptive
    b. Norplant implant
    c. Depo-Provera injection
    d. intrauterine device (IUD)
    e. male condom
    f. female condom
    g. diaphragm
    h. cervical cap
    i. spermicide
    j. Fertility Awareness Method
    k. abstinence
    l. female sterilization
    m. male sterilization

4. Describe the correct procedure for using each of the above-named methods of contraception.

5. Explain how each of the above-named methods of birth control works.

6. Differentiate between failure rate and continuation rate.

7. Evaluate the risks versus the benefits of oral contraceptive use.

8. Explain why male sterilization is considered preferable to female sterilization.

9. Compare and contrast the consequences of not using contraception for a sexually active man with the consequences for a sexually active woman.

10. Identify the criteria that are recommended to guide one's selection of contraceptive method.

TERMINOLOGY

You should be able to define the following key terms:

abortifacient
abstinence
barrier method
Bikini Condom
Billings method
calendar method
cervical cap
circumcise
conception
continuation rate
contraception
contraceptive failure rate
contraceptive immunization
contraceptive
Copper T-380A
corpus luteum
Depo-Provera
diaphragm
douche
ejaculation
estrogen
female condom
fertility
fertility awareness method (FAM)
gossypol
hysterectomy
injectable microspheres
intrauterine device (IUD)
laparoscopy
Levonorgestral

luteinizing hormone-releasing
    hormone (LHRH)
male condom
male contraceptives
mucus-method
Norplant implant
oral contraceptive (OC)
oviducts
ovulation
Pap test
Paragard
pelvic inflammatory disease (PID)
Progstasert
progesterone
prostaglandins
Reality female condom
reversible contraceptives
reversible sterilization
RU 486
sexually transmitted disease
spermicide
sterilization
temperature method
testosterone enanthate
toxic shock syndrome (TSS)
tubal sterilization
vaginal ring
vasa deferentia
vasectomy

MAJOR POINTS/ISSUES

1. People have been seeking ways to prevent pregnancy for thousands of years, and the search for the ideal contraceptive continues today.

2. Because preventing unintended pregnancy and sexually transmitted diseases is crucial to optimal health, decisions about sexual behavior and contraception are among the most significant people can make.

3. A variety of approaches have been used to prevent conception, including barrier methods, hormonal methods, surgical methods, and natural methods.

4. The choice of a contraceptive method depends on effectiveness, convenience, cost, reversibility, side effects and risk factors, and protection against sexually transmitted diseases as well as the method's acceptability in terms of religious or other philosophical beliefs.

5. The oral contraceptive (birth control pill) is a hormonal method of contraception that prevents ovulation, hinders the movement of sperm, and/or affects the uterine lining so that implantation is inhibited.

6. Oral contraceptives are contraindicated for women with a history of heart disease, stroke, cancer, or liver tumor or impaired liver function.

7. The Norplant implant consists of six hormone-filled capsules that are inserted under the skin. It is the most effective reversible contraceptive method known and provides protection for up to five years.

8. Depo-Provera injections contain a long-acting progestin that protects against pregnancy for a period of about three months.

9. The intrauterine device (IUD) is a small plastic object placed in the uterus to prevent pregnancy. Use of the IUD has greatly declined in the United States because most manufacturers have stopped distribution in the face of increased lawsuits associated with complications experienced by IUD users.

10. The male condom, a sheath designed to cover the penis during sexual intercourse is the most popular barrier method of contraception; condom use has increased dramatically, partly because of effectiveness against sexually transmitted diseases. Condoms need to be used exactly as directed during each act of intercourse in order to ensure a high rate of effectiveness.

11. Female condoms consist of a polyurethane or latex sheath that is inserted into the vagina.

12. The diaphragm is a contraceptive device that covers the cervix and blocks sperm from entering. Although use of the diaphragm, which requires a prescription and careful fitting by a medical professional, has declined considerably since oral contraceptives became widely available, it still offers advantages that are important to some couples.

13. The cervical cap is a rubber or plastic cup that adheres to the cervix through suction. It works similarly to the diaphragm.

14. Vaginal spermicides come in the form of foams, creams, jellies, and suppositories. They must be inserted less than one-half hour before intercourse.

15. Abstinence may be chosen to avoid pregnancy and STDs or because of personal needs.

16. The Fertility Awareness Method, a natural method of contraception, is based on avoiding coitus during fertile days of a woman's menstrual cycle. The fertile period can be estimated using the calendar method, the basal body temperature method, and/or the mucus method.

17. Combining methods can increase contraceptive effectiveness and STD protection.

18. Sterilization, the most commonly used method of birth control in the United States, provides complete protection from pregnancy and, although reversible in some cases, should be considered permanent.

19. Vasectomy—male sterilization—involves severing the vasa deferentia in a surgical procedure usually performed in a physician's office.

20. Tubal ligation—female sterilization—involves severing or blocking the oviducts so that the egg cannot reach the uterus.

21. Opinions on when to begin having sexual relations vary from one decade to another and from one group to another.

22. The consequences of not using contraception are markedly different for men and women. Additionally, because women face more serious long-term effects from sexually transmitted diseases, condom use is a more important issue for women.

23. Every sexually active person needs to make a choice about contraception—not choosing anything is the one method known not to work. Issues to be considered in choosing a contraceptive include individual health risks of each method, importance of effectiveness in terms of implications of unwanted pregnancy, possible risk of sexually transmitted diseases, convenience and comfort of the method as viewed by each partner, type of relationship, cost and ease of maintaining each method, and acceptability in terms of religious or philosophical beliefs.

SAMPLE TEST QUESTIONS

Completion

1. Hormonal methods are designed to prevent conception by preventing

    _____.

2. _____ methods of contraception physically prevent the sperm from reaching the egg.

3. The contraceptive characteristic that is perhaps most important to a contraceptive user who eventually wants to have children is _____.

4. The two ingredients in oral contraceptives that prevent ovulation are

    _____ and _____.

5. Norplant implants and Depo-Provera injections contain a synthetic hormone called _____.

6. _____ is a reversible contraceptive method that is contraindicated for women who have never had children.

7. The _____ is the most popular method of barrier contraception.

8. Diaphragms must be left in place for at least _____ hours after intercourse.

9. The male sterilization process is called _____.

10. The Reality brand female condom is made from _____.

True or False

1. The active ingredients in oral contraceptives are progesterone and testosterone.

2. Pap tests are recommended for women who begin taking contraceptives because contraceptives may temporarily increase a woman's susceptibility to some STDs.

3. Norplant is the most effective reversible contraceptive currently available.

4. A postcoital regimen to prevent pregnancy is widely available in other parts of the world but has yet to be approved by the U.S. Food and Drug Administration.

5. Spontaneous expulsion of the IUD is its major disadvantage. It occurs in about 40% of women who have not had children.

6. The most common "failure" of condoms is actually nonuse: taking a chance by using the condom only part of the time.

7. The "Bikini Condom" resembles a string bikini with a pouch that is inserted in the vagina.

8. A cervical cap should be left in place for 72 hours following intercourse.

9. The unfertilized egg lives for about 24 hours.

10. The surgical risks associated with female and male sterilization are about equal.

Multiple Choice

1. Which of the following should be used as a lubricant with condoms?
   a. Vaseline
   b. baby oil
   c. K-Y jelly
   d. butter

2. Most doctors recommend against use of IUDs by young, childless women because:
   a. the risk of serious side effects is higher in this group.
   b. of the potential for irreversibility.
   c. pain during intercourse may occur.
   d. all of the above

3. Which of the following is the LEAST accurate statement about Norplant implants?
   a. Its popularity has dropped recently due to lawsuits.
   b. There are fewer contraindications for using Norplant implants than oral contraceptives.
   c. The menstrual cycle often becomes more regular after one year of Norplant use.
   d. The initial cost associated with the insertion of Norplant implants is low.

4. The Norplant implant:
   a. is a barrier contraceptive
   b. is widely available in the U.S.
   c. was developed in China more than 10 years ago
   d. is used by female and male patients

5. Which of the following is NOT a potential disadvantage of oral contraceptives?
   a. difficult reversibility
   b. depression
   c. weight gain
   d. migraine headaches

6. Oral contraceptive use is contraindicated for women who have a history of:
   a. blood clots
   b. any form of cancer
   c. impaired liver function
   d. all of the above

7. Depo-Provera is administered:
   a. by skin patch
   b. by injection
   c. by implantation
   d. orally

8. The contraceptive mechanism of oral contraceptives is:
   a. creating a sperm barrier
   b. spontaneous abortion
   c. preventing ovulation
   d. unknown

9. The MOST common side effect of intrauterine devices is:
   a. limited reversibility
   b. abnormal menstrual bleeding
   c. occasional painful intercourse
   d. weight gain

10. The method of contraception that is MOST popular among unmarried women in the United States is:
    a. IUDs
    b. oral contraceptives
    c. Norplant implants
    d. spermicides

SAMPLE TEST QUESTIONS ANSWER KEY

Completion

1. ovulation (p. 138)
2. Barrier (p. 138)
3. reversibility (p. 134)
4. progesterone, estrogen (p. 134)
5. progestin (pp. 136–137)
6. Intrauterine device (p. 139)
7. male condom (p. 140)
8. six (p. 144)
9. vasectomy (p. 150)
10. polyurethane (p. 142)

True or False

1. F (p. 134)
2. T (pp. 135–136)
3. T (p. 150)
4. F (pp. 153–156)
5. F (p. 139)
6. T (p. 141)
7. T (p. 143)
8. F (p. 145)
9. T (p. 148)
10. F (p. 149)

Multiple Choice

1. c (p. 140)
2. a (p. 139)
3. d (p. 137)
4. b (p. 137)
5. a (pp. 135–136)
6. d (p. 135)
7. b (pp. 137–138)
8. c (p. 134)
9. b (p. 139)
10. b (p. 135)

Turn to the back of the Study Guide, and complete Wellness Worksheets 28–29.

Chapter 7
Abortion

LEARNING OBJECTIVES

As a result of reading Chapter 7 in the textbook and completing the activities in this Study Guide, you should be able to do the following:

1. Describe the history and current legal status of abortion in the United States.

2. Explain the current debate over abortion, including the main points of the pro-choice and pro-life points of view.

3. Describe the methods of abortion available in the United States.

4. List possible physical and psychological effects of abortion.

5. Discuss the decision-making process a woman and her partner may go through when facing an unintended pregnancy.

TERMINOLOGY

You should be able to define the following key terms:

abortifacient
abortion
amniotic sac
dilation and evacuation (D & E)
Freedom of Access to Clinic Entrance Act
general anesthetic
immune globulin
local anesthetic
menstrual extraction
miscarriage (spontaneous abortion)
Planned Parenthood of Southeastern Pennsylvania v. Casey
pro-choice
pro-life
quickening
regional anesthetic
Roe v. Wade
RU-486
vacuum aspiration
Webster v. Reproductive Health Services

MAJOR POINTS/ISSUES

1. Until the mid-1800s, abortion in the United States was legal before the twentieth week of pregnancy. During the late 1800s, concerns regarding medical control of abortion, "the corruption of women's morals," and use of abortion for birth control resulted in anti-abortion laws in virtually all states. Courts began to invalidate anti-abortion laws in the 1960s on the grounds of constitutional vagueness and violation of right to privacy.

2. The 1973 *Roe v. Wade* Supreme Court case devised new standards to govern abortion decisions. In the first trimester, abortion decisions were left to the judgment of the pregnant woman; in the second trimester, similar rights remained but the state could regulate factors that might protect the health of the woman; in the third trimester, the state could regulate and even prevent all abortions except those considered necessary to preserve the mother's life or health.

3. In the 1989 *Webster v. Reproductive Health Services* Supreme Court case, the Court let stand restrictions on abortion imposed in Missouri and rejected the trimester framework of *Roe v. Wade*. This decision has shifted the political focus of the abortion issue to the states, where great differences in laws and possible discrimination in health care are anticipated.

4. In the 1992 *Planned Parenthood of Southeastern Pennsylvania v. Casey* case, the Court upheld a woman's basic right to abortion and simultaneously gave the state powers to regulate abortion throughout pregnancy, as long as it does not impose "undue burden" on women seeking abortion.

5. The abortion issue has become a major political issue in the United States. The controversy between pro-life and pro-choice movements centers on the issue of when life begins. Pro-life groups believe that a fertilized egg is a human life from the moment of conception and that any abortion is a murder. Pro-choice groups distinguish between stages of fetal development and argue that preserving a woman's right to live her life as she chooses is important and can supersede the rights of the fetus in early stages of development.

6. Overall public opinion in the United States supports legal abortion, although individual opinions change depending on circumstances.

7. A woman considering abortion needs to think about her own religious and moral beliefs, her long-range feelings, the support she has available from others, and the availability and cost of the procedure.

8. The woman who decides against abortion needs to consider decisions about keeping the child, the possibility of single parenthood or marriage, or choosing adoption.

9. RU-486, an abortion pill, causes the uterine lining to shed any fertilized eggs.

10. Methods of abortion include menstrual extraction, vacuum aspiration, dilation and evacuation, saline instillation, and prostaglandins.

11. Abortion complications can include both physical and psychological effects. The overall incidence of problems is significantly reduced with good patient care, early timing of abortion, use of the suction method and local anesthesia, performance by a well-trained clinician, and availability and use of prompt follow-up care.

12. The risk of postabortion complications is low.

13. Some women (especially young women) respond to a possible pregnancy with denial, ascribing the signs of pregnancy to other causes. This delay in confirmation of the pregnancy is a major cause of late abortions, which are associated with more complications.

14. The response of a woman's partner can have a significant influence on how she experiences an unintended pregnancy. Partners can be helpful in weighing important considerations and helping with the chosen course of action.

15. Although a woman's unplanned pregnancy may be stressful for her parents, parents may also be a significant source of support.

16. More than 50% of pregnancies among American women are unintended; many of these are terminated by abortion.

SAMPLE TEST QUESTIONS

Completion

1. In the early years of American history, abortion was widely accepted until the point in the pregnancy marked by _____.

2. The Supreme Court decision that gave the states further powers to regulate abortion as long as they do not impose an "undue burden" on women seeking the procedure was _____.

3. The group that considers abortion wrong in any circumstances is called _____.

4. The primary criterion considered by the Supreme Court in 1973 in *Roe v. Wade* was fetal _____.

5. As a result of legalization and increased access to abortion in the 1970s, the number of late-term abortions went _____.

6. The drug RU-486 blocks the uterine absorption of _____, causing the shedding of the uterine lining and the fertilized egg.

7. An agent or substance that produces abortions is a/an _____.

8. The common name for the generic drug mifepristone is _____.

9. Vacuum aspiration is also known as _____.

10. The most common abortion technique immediately after the 12th week of pregnancy is _____.

True or False

1. Abortion and miscarriage are the same.

2. The case of *Webster v. Reproductive Health Services* legalized abortion.

3. The annual abortion rate has increased steadily every year since 1973.

4. Studies of parental notification laws in Mississippi and Massachusetts found that the parental consent requirement has little effect on the abortion rate among minors.

5. The dilation and evacuation procedure may be performed under a local, regional, or general anesthesia.

6. Subsequent to abortion, over-the-counter medications recommended to relieve minor pain include aspirin or ibuprofen.

7. The risk of mortality in connection with abortion is high and has remained so despite its legalization in 1973.

8. A significant risk of abortion is impaired mental health and severe guilt.

9. The preferred method of abortion up to the 12th week of pregnancy is vacuum aspiration.

10. Adoptions are ordinarily final immediately after all the paperwork is signed.

Multiple Choice

1. In the early years of American history, abortions were commonly permitted up to the _____ week of pregnancy.
   a. 16th
   b. 20th
   c. 24th
   d. 28th

2. The U.S. Supreme Court made a decision in *Roe v. Wade* in _____.
   a. 1973
   b. 1977
   c. 1981
   d. 1994

3. The pro-life position argues that:
   a. women ought to have the right to abortion under any circumstances
   b. abortion ought to be permitted up to the sixth week of pregnancy
   c. abortions are morally wrong
   d. physicians should determine whether a woman may receive an abortion

4. What percent of abortions that occur after the first trimester are performed on teens?
   a. 5%
   b. 10%
   c. 25%
   d. 35%

5. The effect of parental notification laws in Mississippi and Massachusetts has been:
   a. a reduction in abortion rates
   b. little or no change in abortion rates
   c. an increase in abortion rates
   d. difficult to determine

6. The abortion pill is also known as:
   a. RU-486
   b. DC pill
   c. DE pill
   d. prosteglandins pill

7. RU-486 has the generic name:
   a. prosteglandins
   b. abortifacients
   c. mifepristone
   d. sulfacetamide

8. The abortion method preferred shortly after the first missed period is:
   a. menstrual extraction
   b. vacuum aspiration
   c. dilation and evacuation
   d. dilation and curettage

9. Recommended OTC pain medication after abortion is:
   a. aspirin
   b. Advil
   c. Motrin
   d. acetaminophen

10. The MOST accurate statement regarding adoption is:
    a. Adoption is final once all paperwork is completed and a court approves the adoption.
    b. Adoption agencies are essentially adoption brokers whose clients are potential adoptive parents.
    c. Adoption agencies and adoptive parents often give financial help to birth mothers.
    d. State laws are uniform regarding adoption.

SAMPLE TEST QUESTIONS ANSWER KEY

Completion

1. "quickening" (p. 164)
2. *Planned Parenthood of Southeastern Pennsylvania v. Casey* (p. 164)
3. "pro-life" (p. 165)
4. viability (p. 164)
5. down (p. 170)
6. progesterone (p. 174)
7. abortifacients (p. 172)
8. RU-486 (p. 174)
9. suction curettage (p. 174)
10. dilation and evacuation (p. 174)

True or False

1. F (p. 164)
2. F (p. 164)
3. F (p. 165)
4. T (p. 170)
5. T (p. 174)
6. F (p. 176)
7. F (p. 176)
8. F (p. 176)
9. T (p. 174)
10. F (p. 171)

Multiple Choice

1. b (p. 164)
2. a (p. 164)
3. c (p. 165)
4. d (p. 169)
5. b (p. 170)
6. a (p. 174)
7. c (p. 174)
8. a (p. 174)
9. d (p. 176)
10. c (p. 171)

Turn to the back of the Study Guide, and complete Wellness Worksheets 30–31.

Chapter 8
Pregnancy and Childbirth

LEARNING OBJECTIVES

As a result of reading Chapter 8 in the textbook and completing the activities in this Study Guide, you should be able to do the following:

1. Identify key issues to consider when deciding about becoming a parent.

2. Explain the process of conception.

3. Describe the most common causes and treatments for infertility.

4. Describe the physical and emotional changes that a pregnant woman typically experiences.

5. Discuss the stages of fetal development.

6. Identify the important elements of good prenatal care.

7. Describe the process of labor and delivery.

TERMINOLOGY

You should be able to define the following key terms:

afterbirth	Down syndrome
alpha-fetoprotein (AFP) screening	eclampsia
amniocentesis	ectopic pregnancy
amniotic fluid	ejaculation
amniotic sac	electronic fetal monitoring (EFM)
Apgar score	embryo
artificial (intrauterine) insemination	endometriosis
attachment	endometrium
blastocyst	episiotomy
Braxton Hicks contractions	false labor
cervix	fertilization
cesarean section	fertilized egg (zygote)
chorionic villi	fetal alcohol syndrome (FAS)
chorionic villus sampling (CVS)	fetus
chromosomes	folic acid
colostrum	follicle
conception	fraternal twins
congenital malformation	gamete intrafallopian transfer (GIFT)
contraction	gene
crowning	genetic code

genetic counselors
Hegar's sign
human chorionic gonadotropin (HCG)
identical twins
immunities
in vitro fertilization (IVF)
infant mortality
infertility
intrauterine insemination
Kegel exercises
labor
lactation
lightening
lochia
low birth weight (LBW)
ovary
oviduct (fallopian tube)
placenta
postpartum depression
postpartum period
preconception care
preeclampsia
pregnancy
pregnancy tests

prenatal care
prenatal testing
prepared childbirth
Rh incompatibilities
rooming-in
seminal vesicles
sonogram
sperm cells
spontaneous abortion (miscarriage)
sudden infant death syndrome (SIDS)
surrogate motherhood
teratogen
testis
thalidomide
toxemia
transition
trimester
ultrasonography
umbilical cord
urethra
uterus
vagina
vasa deferentia
zygote intrafallopian transfer (ZIFT)

MAJOR POINTS/ISSUES

1. Today it is possible to choose whether, when, and how to have a child; it is also possible to make choices in young adulthood that will help keep all options open for the day one is ready to have a child.

2. There are many factors to consider when deciding if and when to have a child. Those factors include physical health and age, financial circumstances, relationship with partner, educational, career and child-care plans, emotional readiness for parenthood, social support system, personal qualities, attitudes toward children, aptitude for parenting, and philosophical beliefs.

3. Preconception care can reduce risks for both mother and child; it typically involves examination of such factors as preexisting medical conditions, current medications, past history of pregnancy, age of the mother, lifestyle behaviors, infections, nutritional status, and family history of genetic disease.

4. Pregnancy begins with a complex process wherein one sperm penetrates the membrane of one egg (fertilization) and culminates with the birth, after about nine months' gestation, of the baby.

5. Together the egg and sperm carry the genetic code, a set of instructions for development, which provides the blueprint for a new and unique person.

6. Infertility is a serious problem for about 8% of couples in the United States. Many infertility problems are treatable through surgery, fertility drugs, or more advanced techniques like artificial insemination and in vitro fertilization. Nearly half of the factors contributing to infertility are male; 15% of cases are due to problems of both partners.

7. Some treatments for infertility are expensive, emotionally draining, and have limited success rates.

8. One way to avoid some forms of infertility is to protect oneself against STDs and to get immediate treatment for any diseases contracted. Pelvic inflammatory disease is especially threatening to female fertility.

9. Early recognition of pregnancy, through recognition of common signs and symptoms, is important, especially for women with physical problems and/or nutritional deficiencies. Early pregnancy tests detect the presence of human chorionic gonadotropin in the urine or blood of the mother.

10. During pregnancy, significant changes occur throughout the woman's body to accommodate the growing fetus and in preparation for childbirth and breastfeeding.

11. Pregnancy is divided into trimesters based on fetal development. As the fertilized egg divides, its outer cells develop into the placenta, umbilical cord, and amniotic sac. Fetal anatomy is almost completely formed in the first trimester and is refined in the second; needed fats and pounds are added during the third trimester.

12. A variety of prenatal tests are now available that can provide information about genetic abnormalities, size, and gender.

13. Adequate prenatal care includes good nutrition; regular physical activity; avoiding drugs, alcohol, tobacco, infections, and other harmful agents or conditions; limiting caffeine consumption; childbirth classes; and regular medical checkups.

14. It is estimated that 10 to 40% of pregnancies end with a miscarriage; most of these occur during the first trimester of pregnancy and may not even be recognized by the woman.

15. Ectopic pregnancy, implantation of a fertilized egg in the oviduct or in another location outside the uterus, can be dangerous because it can result in internal bleeding and/or infertility. Spontaneous abortion, toxemia, and low birth weight are other potential complications of pregnancy.

16. A wide variety of childbirth choices is now available to prospective parents. Positive outcomes are most likely if the parents make an informed choice based on what feels most comfortable for them.

17. Alternative birth centers, certified nurse-midwives, and home births provide options to more traditional methods of childbirth. These options, each with their own advantages and disadvantages, should be available for consideration to all birthing women.

18. The process of childbirth includes three stages: first, the contractions that open the cervix and cause the baby to descend; second, the actual birth of the baby; third, the delivery of the placenta.

19. During the postpartum period, the mother's body begins to return to its prepregnancy state, and she may begin to breastfeed. Some new mothers experience postpartum depression.

20. Cesarean deliveries account for 20% of births. Cesarean sections are major surgeries but are relatively safe.

21. Attachment between parent and child is crucial to the child's social, emotional, and intellectual development. Both mother and father must adjust to their new roles as parents as they develop a strong emotional tie to their child.

SAMPLE TEST QUESTIONS

Completion

1. For middle-class families with two children, it costs about _____ to raise a child to age 18.

2. The process involving the fusion of the sperm and the egg is called

   _____.

3. The woman's egg travels from the ovary to the uterus through the

   _____ tube.

4. The assisted fertilization technique that involves mixing sperm with eggs in a laboratory dish is called _____ fertilization.

5. The earliest tests for pregnancy are chemical tests designed to detect the presence of

   _____.

6. A normal amount of weight gain for a pregnant woman is _____.

7. Preliminary contractions preparing the uterus for childbirth are called _____ contractions.

8. The blastocyst is associated with the _____ trimester of pregnancy.

9. The most rapid period of fetal differentiation occurs during the _____ trimester.

10. The visual image of the fetus created by ultrasound technology is called a/an

    _____.

True or False

1. Almost one third of all U.S. births are to unmarried women.

2. Alpha-fetoprotein (AFP) screening is used to detect the sex of the baby prior to birth.

3. Amniocentesis may be used to detect birth defects.

4. Blood testing is an important part of prenatal care.

5. Moderate alcohol consumption by a pregnant woman is safe for her unborn baby.

6. Cigarette smoking is associated with low birth weight.

7. A pregnant woman may safely consume up to six cups of coffee (or equivalent caffeinated beverages and foods) per day.

8. Kegel exercises are a form of breathing exercise to induce relaxation.

9. An ectopic pregnancy is one in which the fertilized egg implants itself outside the uterus.

10. Preeclampsia is a form of toxicity due to alcohol or drug use.

Multiple Choice

1. Which of the following women are at greater risk from pregnancy based on age?
   a. women under 25
   b. women over 30
   c. women 25–35
   d. teens and women over 35

2. The annual cost of raising a child averages about:
   a. $2500
   b. $5000
   c. $7500
   d. $10,000

3. Toxoplasmosis is MOST likely to be contracted from which of the following house pets?
   a. dogs
   b. cats
   c. birds
   d. fish

4. If an egg is not fertilized it only lasts about _____ hours.
   a. 12
   b. 24
   c. 48
   d. 96

5. Which of the following describes fertilization that occurs in the fallopian tubes?
   a. in vitro fertilization
   b. gamete intrafallopian transfer
   c. zygote intrafallopian transfer
   d. prostaglandins fallopian transfer

6. Pregnancy tests seek to detect:
   a. human chorionic gonadotropin
   b. prostaglandins
   c. estrogen
   d. progesterone

7. Which of the following characterizes pregnancy?
   a. weight loss
   b. reduced respiratory efficiency
   c. narrowing of rib cage
   d. increased blood volume

8. The term "lightening" refers to the:
   a. breaking of the water
   b. fetus sinking in the uterus
   c. discovery of an ectopic pregnancy
   d. commencement of contractions

9. The fertilized egg becomes a fetus:
   a. at conception
   b. in the first trimester
   c. in the second trimester
   d. in the third trimester

10. Pregnant women who are HIV positive have approximately a/an _____ chance of transmitting HIV to their unborn babies if they do not receive any prophylactic treatment.
    a. 8%
    b. 10%
    c. 25%
    d. 100%

SAMPLE TEST QUESTIONS ANSWER KEY

Completion

1. $138,000 (p. 184)
2. conception (p. 187)
3. fallopian (p. 188)
4. in vitro (p. 191)
5. human chorionic gonadotropin (p. 193)
6. 18–25% (p. 194)
7. Braxton Hicks (p. 194)
8. first (p. 195)
9. first (p. 196)
10. sonogram (p. 198)

True or False

1. T (p. 184)
2. F (p. 199)
3. T (pp. 198–199)
4. T (p. 200)
5. F (p. 200)
6. T (p. 200)
7. F (p. 202)
8. F (p. 203)
9. T (p. 204)
10. F (p. 205)

Multiple Choice

1. a (p. 185)
2. c (p. 184)
3. b (p. 185)
4. b (p. 188)
5. b (p. 191)
6. a (p. 192)
7. d (p. 194)
8. b (p. 194)
9. b (p. 197)
10. c (p. 202)

Turn to the back of the Study Guide, and complete Wellness Worksheets 32–35.

Chapter 9
The Use and Abuse of Psychoactive Drugs

LEARNING OBJECTIVES

As a result of reading Chapter 9 in the textbook and completing the activities in this Study Guide, you should be able to do the following:

1. Define and discuss the concepts of addictive behavior, substance abuse, and substance dependence.

2. Explain factors contributing to drug use and dependence.

3. List the major categories of psychoactive drugs and describe their effects.

4. Describe the primary ways psychoactive drugs are introduced into the body.

5. Discuss the potential for abuse of and dependence on psychoactive drugs.

6. Discuss the social issues related to psychoactive drug use.

7. Describe the primary approaches to preventing and treating drug abuse.

8. Evaluate the role of drugs and other addictive behaviors in your life, and identify your personal risk for abusing drugs and becoming dependent upon them.

TERMINOLOGY

You should be able to define the following key terms:

absorption
addiction
addictive behavior
altered states of consciousness
amphetamine ("uppers," "speed")
anesthetic
antidepressants (Elavil, Tofranil, Prozac)
asphyxiation
attention deficit disorder
"bad trip" ("bummer")
barbiturate
benzodiazepines (Xanax, Valium, Librium)
biochemical
Cannabis sativa (Indian hemp plant)
central nervous system (CNS)
"China White"
chromosomes

cocaine ("coke," "snow")
cocaine-affected babies (crack babies)
codeine
codependency
compulsive use
crack
cross-tolerance
cumulative effects
deliriants
delirium
dependence (dependency)
depersonalization
depressant
depression
designer drugs
dextroamphetamine (Dexedrine)
diazepam (Valium)

dimethosy-methylamphetamine (STP)
dimethyltryptamine (DMT)
dose-response function
dronabinol
drug
drug abuse
drug dependence
drug interactions
drug legalization
drug testing
drug substitution programs
drug use
drugs
DTs
dual disorder
endorphins
ephedrine
escalation
euphoria
flashback
"free-basing"
hallucinogen
hashish
heroin
high
"ice"
ingestion
inhalant
inhalation
injecting drug use
injection
insomnia
intoxication
intramuscular
intravenous (IV, mainline)
LAAM
lithium salts
lysergic acid diethylamide (LSD)
mania
manic-depressive disorder
marijuana
MDMA (ecstasy)
meperidine
mescaline (peyote)
methadone
methamphetamine (Methedrine)
methaqualone (Quaalude)
method of use
morphine

Narcotics Anonymous
opioid
overdose
panic reaction
paranoid behavior
parkinsonism
pathological
pharmacological properties
pharmacology
pharmacy
phencyclidine (PCP, "angel dust,"
    "hog," "peace pill")
phobias
physical dependence
physical tolerance
placebo
placebo effect
prescription
proprioception
psilocybin
psychedelics (hallucinogens)
psychoactive drug
psychosis
reinforcement
respiratory collapse
schizophrenia
sedation
sedative-hypnotic
seizures
self-help programs
setting
"snorting"
"speedball" mixtures
state dependence
sterilization
stimulant
subcutaneous
substance abuse
substance dependence
synesthesia
tetrahydrocannabinol (THC)
therapeutic community
time-action function
tolerance
tranquilizer
treatment centers
vasoconstriction
withdrawal

Major Points and Issues

1. The use of drugs for both medical and social purposes is widespread in American society.

2. Addiction is not limited to drug use. People may be addicted to gambling, use of the Internet, spending money, or even exercise.

3. Drug abuse is characterized by social or academic failure due to drug use, putting one's self at risk, legal problems, and continuing social and interpersonal problems made worse by drug use.

4. Drug dependence is more complex than drug use and is defined by physical tolerance, withdrawal, increasing dosages, expressed desire to quit using drugs, investing disproportionate time and energy in getting drugs, reducing or eliminating social contacts due to drug use, and continuing use after recognizing a problem with drug use.

5. People use drug's for a wide variety of personal, social, and environmental reasons.

6. A drug's effect on the body is determined by many factors including dose, duration of drug use, method of use, a user's personal characteristics, including expectations, and the social setting in which the drug is used.

7. In this chapter drugs are divided into six groups: opioids, central nervous system depressants, central nervous system stimulants, marijuana, hallucinogens, and inhalants.

8. The social and economic cost of drug use and abuse is high. Enforcement, prevention efforts, and treatment all consume many resources. The personal cost to families and individuals is also high and difficult to calculate in financial terms.

9. There are conflicting views about drug use and abuse. Some people recommend the legalization of some drugs, such as marijuana and heroin, while others prefer more restrictions and argue for more aggressive use of drug testing to identify drug users.

10. Drug treatment approaches vary and include drug substitution programs, self-help groups, and medical detoxification.

SAMPLE TEST QUESTIONS

Completion

1. The drugs most frequently associated with abuse are _____ drugs.

2. The proportion of the population that used drugs was at its highest in approximately the year _____.

3. Tolerance and withdrawal are two of seven specific criteria that define drug _____.

4. People with psychiatric illness are _____ likely to suffer from drug dependency.

5. A drug's overall effects on a person's body chemistry, behavior, and psychology are its _____ properties.

6. The relationship between the amount of a drug taken and the intensity of the drug effect is the _____ relationship.

7. If an individual received an inert substance but responded to it as if it were an active drug, that would be an example of the _____ effect.

8. Of the six categories of drugs identified in this chapter, the _____ are the only group of drugs that are narcotics.

9. Addictive behaviors are habits that are _____.

10. The most widely used psychoactive drug in the United States is _____.

True or False

1. LSD has been used in the past by psychiatrists to facilitate discussions about repressed feelings.

2. The intoxicating effects of DMT and STP both last longer than LSD.

3. Mescaline is a ceremonial drug of the Native North American Church.

4. Inhalants are very popular among American teens. Nearly 20% of all twelfth graders have used inhalants.

5. The personal and family costs of drug abuse are high but the financial costs are low.

6. More than 20,000 Americans die annually due to drug abuse.

7. The text suggests that as many as 10% of the American work force uses drugs.

8. Most drug testing involves the use of a breathalyzer.

9. Drug substitution programs are losing favor because of their relatively high cost.

10. Heroin and other injectable drugs are responsible for much of the HIV infection in America.

Multiple Choice

1. The drugs MOST frequently associated with drug abuse are:
   a. over-the-counter drugs
   b. prescription drugs
   c. psychoactive drugs
   d. appetite suppression drugs

2. Which characteristic is MOST closely associated with the historical definition of addiction?
   a. physical tolerance
   b. habitual use
   c. increased use
   d. disease

3. Contemporary characteristics of addiction include:
   a. compulsion
   b. loss of control
   c. drug use escalation
   d. all of the above

4. Which of the following has the potential for addiction?
   a. drug use
   b. spending money
   c. Internet use
   d. all of the above

5. After 1900, the peak of recreational drug use in this country occurred in:
   a. 1959
   b. 1969
   c. 1979
   d. 1989

6. Drug dependence is characterized by:
   a. recurrent use
   b. drug-related legal problems
   c. withdrawal symptoms
   d. interpersonal and social problems caused by drug use

7. The characteristic LEAST predictive of drug use is:
   a. exposure to drug use
   b. children of single mothers who did not complete high school
   c. risk-taking personality
   d. ethnicity

8. The relationship between the amount of a drug taken and its effects is the:
   a. time-action function
   b. time-response function
   c. dose-action function
   d. dose-response function

9. The placebo effect is:
   a. a pharmacological property
   b. the product of believing in an inert substance
   c. worthless
   d. increased by the dose of administered substance

10. Which of the following categories of drugs are narcotics?
    a. central nervous system depressants
    b. central nervous system stimulants
    c. opioids
    d. cannabis products

SAMPLE TEST QUESTIONS ANSWER KEY

Completion

1. psychoactive (p. 216)
2. 1900 (p. 219)
3. dependence (p. 221)
4. more (p. 223)
5. pharmacological (p. 223)
6. dose-response (p. 224)
7. placebo (p. 226)
8. opioids (p. 227)
9. out of control (p. 216)
10. marijuana (p. 231)

True or False

1. T (p. 233)
2. F (p. 233)
3. T (p. 233)
4. T (p. 234)
5. F (p. 234)
6. T (p. 235)
7. T (p. 235)
8. F (p. 236)
9. F (p. 236)
10. T (p. 225)

Multiple Choice

1. c (p. 216)
2. a (p. 216)
3. d (pp. 216–217
4. d (p. 217)
5. c (p. 219)
6. c (p. 221)
7. d (p. 221)
8. d (p. 224)
9. b (p. 226)
10. c (p. 277)

Turn to the back of the Study Guide, and complete Wellness Worksheets 36–38.

Chapter 10
The Responsible Use of Alcohol

LEARNING OBJECTIVES

As a result of reading Chapter 10 in the textbook and completing the activities in this Study Guide, you should be able to do the following:

1. Define the nature and characteristics of alcohol.

2. Explain how alcohol is absorbed and metabolized by the body.

3. Describe the immediate and long-term effects of drinking alcohol.

4. Identify the potential health benefits of alcohol consumption.

5. Define alcohol abuse, binge drinking, and alcoholism, and discuss their effects on the drinker and others.

6. Define the relationships between alcohol abuse and gender and ethnicity.

7. Discuss approaches to treatment of alcohol abuse and alcoholism.

8. Evaluate the role of alcohol in your life, and list strategies for using it responsibly, including being a responsible role model for people in your peer group.

TERMINOLOGY

You should be able to define the following key terms:

absorption
acetaldehyde
addiction
alcohol
alcohol absorption
alcohol abuse
alcohol dependence
alcohol metabolism
alcohol poisoning
Alcoholics Anonymous
alcoholism
binge drinking
blood alcohol concentration (BAC)
cardiac myopathy
central nervous system depressant
cirrhosis of the liver

codependent
distillation
disulfiram (Antabuse)
dose-response relationship
DTs (delirium tremens)
ethyl alcohol
fermented
fetal alcohol syndrome (FAS)
fortified wines
hallucination
"hangover"
high-density lipoprotein (HDL)
intoxication
isopropyl alcohol
metabolism
naltrexone

paranoia
proof value
sedate
sobriety
stimulant

stupor
testicular atrophy
tolerance
withdrawal
zero tolerance

MAJOR POINTS/ISSUES

1. Although alcohol has long been a part of human celebrations, it is a drug capable of causing addiction and harmful physiological effects.

2. Ethyl alcohol is the psychoactive ingredient in alcoholic beverages.

3. Alcohol concentration in a beverage is indicated by proof value, which is defined as two times the percentage concentration.

4. How long it takes alcohol to be absorbed into the bloodstream from the stomach depends on the amount, type, and proof of the beverage, the time taken to drink it, and whether there is food in the stomach. The body weight and composition and gender of the drinker are also important factors that influence the time and degree of intoxication.

5. After alcohol is absorbed into the bloodstream, it is distributed throughout the body. As alcohol is circulated through the liver, it is metabolized at the rate of about 0.3 to 0.5 ounces per hour, depending on body weight and other factors.

6. A small percentage of alcohol is not metabolized by the liver but excreted unchanged via the lungs, kidneys, and sweat glands. This is the basis for breath and urine analyses to determine alcohol levels.

7. The blood alcohol content will remain low as long as a person drinks less alcohol per hour than the amount he or she can metabolize in an hour.

8. Women generally have higher BACs than men who drink the same amount.

9. Alcohol in low doses acts on people to reduce their inhibitions, which is often interpreted as helping one relax and feel more at ease. In social settings, alcohol often seems to act like a stimulant, but alcohol is actually a central nervous system depressant.

10. At higher concentrations, alcohol interferes with motor coordination, verbal performance, and intellectual functions. Alcohol affects internal body temperature, changes sleep patterns, and has an adverse effect on sexual performance. High doses can result in coma and death.

11. Acute alcohol poisoning occurs frequently and can cause death.

12. Combining alcohol with other drugs is a life-threatening behavior. The combined effects are often greater than the sum of their individual effects.

13. Over half of all traffic fatalities are associated with alcohol use. There is a dose-response relationship between the amount of alcohol consumed and the risk of auto crashes.

14. Chronic use of alcohol is associated with cirrhosis of the liver, cardiac problems, and certain cancers. On the average, alcohol abusers live 10 to 12 years less than nonabusers.

15. Any alcohol ingested by a pregnant woman crosses the placenta into the circulation of the fetus. Women who drink alcohol are putting their babies at risk for fetal alcohol syndrome (FAS), a collection of serious birth defects. Since no safe level of alcohol has been identified for pregnant women, abstinence is the safest course.

16. Signs of alcohol abuse include drinking secretively, using alcohol as a "crutch," feeling uncomfortable without alcohol, increasing average consumption, drinking before driving, drinking at all hours, and getting drunk often.

17. Alcohol dependence, or alcoholism, involves more extensive problems than alcohol abuse, usually involving tolerance or withdrawal.

18. Binge drinking is a common form of alcohol abuse on college campuses. Binge drinkers suffer more academic, legal, and interpersonal problems than students who do not binge drink.

19. There are four common patterns of alcohol abuse: regular daily intake of large amounts, regular heavy drinking limited to weekends, long periods of sobriety interspersed with binges, and heavy drinking limited to periods of stress.

20. People of all ethnic groups and social and economic classes abuse alcohol. The pattern of abuse usually differs between men and women and from one ethnic group to another. It is estimated that about 3% of men and 1% of women are alcoholic.

21. The exact causes of alcoholism are not known. There apparently is a genetic contribution to alcoholism, but other factors, including personality disorders, destructive child-rearing practices, desire to imitate others, urbanization, lack of positive family support, increased mobility, and changing societal values are also part of the picture.

22. Alcohol can harm many different organs and tissues resulting in not only cirrhosis of the liver, but also asthma, gout, diabetes, and recurrent infections.

23. Psychiatric problems involved with alcohol abuse include paranoia, memory loss, and lying.

24. Alcohol abusers come from all socioeconomic classes.

25. Some alcoholics recover without professional help and others participate in a variety of treatment programs. The majority of alcoholics do not stop drinking on their own.

26. A person associated with an alcoholic needs to be careful not to become an enabler; that is, someone who, perhaps unknowingly, allows another to continue excessive use of alcohol.

27. The responsible use of alcohol means keeping the BAC low and behavior always under control. Ways to do so include drinking slowly and spacing drinks, eating before and while drinking, being a responsible host or hostess, having responsible attitudes toward alcohol, and learning about alcohol abuse prevention programs.

28. To make responsible, informed choices about alcohol, it is important to learn whether there is any history of alcohol abuse or alcoholism in the family.

29. Millions of people grow up in alcoholic homes, learning methods of behavior that do not support healthy development. Today the special problems and needs of children of alcoholics (including adult children of alcoholics) are recognized. Support groups and family therapy provide help.

SAMPLE TEST QUESTIONS

Completion

1. The concentration of alcohol in a beverage is indicated by the _____.

2. The main site of alcohol metabolism is the _____.

3. Alcohol is a central nervous system _____.

4. The fact that increased alcohol consumption greatly increases the risk of an auto crash demonstrates the _____ relationship.

5. People who continue drinking after being diagnosed with cirrhosis of the liver have only a _____% chance of surviving five more years.

6. The collection of birth defects that result from a pregnant woman's heavy drinking is known as _____ syndrome.

7. The level of high density lipoproteins, otherwise known as the "good" cholesterol, seems to go _____ as a result of moderate drinking.

8. The medical emergency caused by overdrinking and characterized by disorientation, confusion, seizures, and hallucinations is known as _____.

9. Although many factors affect a person's risk for alcoholism, as much as 50% of the risk is determined by _____ factors.

10. A person who facilitates the alcohol abuse of another person is a/an

_____.

True or False

1. Fortified wines have approximately the same amount of alcohol as all other wines.

2. Blood alcohol concentration is influenced by volume of alcohol consumption only.

3. The rate of alcohol metabolism cannot be accelerated.

4. Drivers are usually safe to drive up to a blood alcohol level of 0.20%.

5. Women usually develop cirrhosis of the liver at higher rates than men.

6. Alcoholics have cancer rates that are approximately 10 times higher than non-drinkers.

7. Binge drinking students engage in many high risk behaviors that occur less frequently in the lives of non-drinking students.

8. Withdrawal is not possible for people who are addicted to alcohol.

9. One way to promote responsible drinking is to hold a drinker accountable for his or her behavior.

10. Children of alcoholics are more likely to become alcoholic and to marry an alcoholic than a member of the general population is.

Multiple Choice

1. About _____ of alcohol is absorbed in the stomach.
   a. 20%
   b. 40%
   c. 60%
   d. 80%

2. Women generally have higher BACs than men because they:
   a. drink more
   b. are less experienced drinkers
   c. have a higher percentage of body fat, which influences metabolism of alcohol
   d. don't eat when they drink

3. _____ atrophy occurs with long-term overuse of alcohol.
   a. Muscular
   b. Testicular
   c. Brain
   d. Lung

4. A primary risk of alcohol poisoning is:
    a. depressed respiration
    b. aspiration of vomit
    c. aspiration of other fluids
    d. all of the above

5. The "zero tolerance" blood alcohol level set in most states is:
    a. 0.00%
    b. 0.02%
    c. 0.08%
    d. 0.10%

6. How many Americans over age 15 drink alcohol?
    a. half
    b. two-thirds
    c. one-fourth
    d. three-fourths

7. All other things being equal, which of the following people is going to get intoxicated most quickly?
    a. 200-lb male
    b. 150-lb female
    c. 150-lb male
    d. 125-lb female

8. Drinking alcohol has all of these physical effects EXCEPT:
    a. promoting sounder sleep
    b. dilating blood vessels
    c. reducing sense of taste
    d. reducing erection response

9. The best way to drink moderately is to:
    a. use carbonated mixers
    b. drink on an empty stomach
    c. drink a 50-proof beverage instead of a 40-proof one
    d. space your drinks out

10. If a beverage is 100 proof, it contains _____% alcohol.
    a. 25
    b. 50
    c. 100
    d. 200

SAMPLE TEST QUESTIONS ANSWER KEY

Completion

1. proof value (p. 248)
2. liver (p. 249)
3. depressant (p. 251)
4. dose-response (p. 253)
5. 50 (p. 254)
6. fetal alcohol (p. 255)
7. up (p. 257)
8. delirium tremens (p. 259)
9. genetic (p. 261)
10. enabler or codependent (p. 264)

True or False

1. F (p. 248)
2. F (p. 249)
3. T (p. 249)
4. F (p. 253)
5. F (p. 254)
6. T (p. 255)
7. T (p. 258)
8. F (p. 259)
9. T (p. 266)
10. T (p. 260)

Multiple Choice

1. a (p. 248)
2. c (p. 249)
3. b (p. 251)
4. d (p. 252)
5. b (p. 253)
6. b (p. 248)
7. d (p. 249)
8. a (p. 251)
9. d (p. 265)
10. b (p. 248)

Turn to the back of the Study Guide, and complete Wellness Worksheets 39–41.

Chapter 11
Toward a Tobacco-Free Society

LEARNING OBJECTIVES

As a result of reading Chapter 11 in the textbook and completing the activities in this Study Guide, you should be able to do the following:

1. List reasons why people start using tobacco and why they continue to use it.

2. Explain the short- and long-term health risks associated with tobacco use.

3. Discuss the effects of environmental tobacco smoke on nonsmokers.

4. Describe the social costs of tobacco, and list actions that have been taken to combat smoking in the public and private sectors.

5. Prepare plans to stop using tobacco and to avoid environmental tobacco smoke.

TERMINOLOGY

You should be able to define the following key terms:

addiction
angina pectoris
aortic aneurysm
asthma
atherosclerosis
benzo(a)pyrene
carbon monoxide
carboxyhemoglobin
carcinogen
cerebral cortex
chicartas
chronic bronchitis
chronic obstructive lung disease (COLD)
cigarette tar
clove cigarettes
cocarcinogen
"cold turkey"
coronary heart disease (CHD)
emphysema
environmental tobacco smoke (ETS)
Fairness Doctrine
formaldehyde
high-density lipoprotein (HDL)
kreteks

low birth weight
lung cancer
macrophages
mainstream smoke
myocardial infarction
myocardium
nicotine
nicotine poisoning
peptic ulcers
plaque
premature birth
psychoactive drug
pulmonary heart disease
respiratory cilia
secondary reinforcers
sidestream smoke
smokeless tobacco
smoking
stroke
sudden infant death syndrome (SIDS)
tobacco
tolerance
withdrawal

MAJOR POINTS AND ISSUES

1. Once considered a very suave behavior, smoking has fallen into disfavor, and many smokers feel badly about their smoking behavior and wish they could quit. Fully 75% of smokers want to quit but find they cannot.

2. Nicotine is a powerful psychoactive drug, and most long-term smokers are addicted. Nicotine's primary attraction seems to be due to its ability to modulate everyday emotions. At low doses nicotine appears to act as a stimulant.

3. Tobacco addiction produces tolerance and withdrawal, and smokers become addicted after a short smoking history.

4. Smoking and other tobacco use start for a variety of reasons including: social encouragement, to combat weight gain, to cope with stress, and to stimulate one's self.

5. Advertising clearly targets youthful potential smokers. Advertising icon Joe Camel is recognized by half of all 3–6-year-olds, and 90% of 6-year-olds associate Joe Camel with smoking. This is in spite of the fact that tobacco advertising has been banned from television and radio for more than 25 years.

6. A variety of circumstances put young people at risk for tobacco use including a smoking parent; smoking siblings; smoking peers; coming from a blue-collar, single-parent, or low-income home; and poor academic performance.

7. Tobacco smoke is poison and includes carcinogens, cocarcinogens, and formaldehyde. Nicotine poisoning symptoms include dizziness, faintness, rapid pulse, cold, clammy skin, nausea, vomiting, and diarrhea.

8. Long-term effects of smoking include cardiovascular disease, respiratory disease, emphysema, lung cancer, and other cancers.

9. Smokeless tobacco, although not as dangerous as smoking, does have health risks, including elevated risk of numerous cancers. Smokeless tobacco use is increasing, especially among young males.

10. Nonsmokers also suffer the effects of smoking if they are exposed to environmental tobacco smoke (ETS). Environmental tobacco smoke is also called sidestream smoke. Infants and children are particularly affected by environmental tobacco smoke.

11. The cost of health care for tobacco-generated health problems is high, exceeding not only the total tax assessed on tobacco but the total amount spent on tobacco.

SAMPLE TEST QUESTIONS

Completion

1. The psychoactive ingredient in tobacco smoke is _____.

2. Activities that smokers associate with smoking are _____ reinforcers.

3. The tobacco advertising icon most easily recognized by young children is _____.

4. Effects of environmental tobacco smoke include coughs, headaches, and _____ irritation.

5. Tobacco smoke ingredients benzo(a)pyrene and urethane are _____.

6. Smoking is strongly related to the buildup of plaques in the coronary artery that results in a type of heart attack called _____.

7. Smoking reduces the amount of _____ cholesterol.

8. The acronym COLD stands for _____.

9. Chronic bronchitis is a precursor of _____ cancer.

10. The major cumulative effect of tobacco use is _____ life expectancy.

True or False

1. Smokers spend far more days sick than nonsmokers.

2. Smokeless tobacco use is increasing as much among young women as young men.

3. Cigar and pipe smokers have equal health risks to cigarette smokers.

4. Clove cigarettes are risk free.

5. Environmental tobacco smoke is also known as mainstream smoke.

6. Infants and children are affected more severely than adults by sidestream smoke.

7. Smoking mothers increase the risk of their children dying from sudden infant death syndrome.

8. The tobacco industry contributes heavily to the political campaigns of representatives who support tobacco industry initiatives.

9. The most effective way to stop smoking is to quit "cold turkey."

10. Tobacco contributes to more deaths annually than alcohol, firearms, illicit drugs, and motor vehicle crashes combined.

Multiple Choice

1. Tobacco products which have experienced the GREATEST increase in popularity in the past five years are:
   a. cigarettes
   b. cigars
   c. chewing tobacco
   d. snuff

2. The chemical in tobacco smoke that creates addiction is:
   a. benzo(a)pyrene
   b. formaldehyde
   c. nicotine
   d. tar

3. Nicotine is associated with which of the following?
   a. loss of control
   b. tolerance
   c. withdrawal
   d. all of the above

4. If a person is able to forgo smoking until the age of _____ , they probably will never start.
   a. 12
   b. 14
   c. 18
   d. 20

5. Anti-smoking messages were required in the national media after 1967 due to the:
   a. FDA Act
   b. OSHA regulations
   c. Fairness Doctrine
   d. Department of Agriculture

6. The group MOST vulnerable to environmental tobacco smoke is:
   a. infants and children
   b. adolescents
   c. mothers
   d. older adults

7. The primary cancer associated with smoking is _____ cancer.
   a. brain
   b. liver
   c. pancreatic
   d. lung

8. When the lungs lose their elasticity the health problem is:
   a. COLD
   b. cancer
   c. emphysema
   d. bronchitis

9. Smokeless tobacco use is increasing MOST among:
   a. adult males
   b. young males
   c. adults females
   d. young females

10. Kreteks is another name for:
    a. smokeless tobacco
    b. clove cigarettes
    c. tobacco cigarettes
    d. cigars

SAMPLE TEST QUESTIONS ANSWER KEY

Completion

1. nicotine (p. 274)
2. secondary (p. 276)
3. Joe Camel (p. 276)
4. eye (p. 286)
5. carcinogens (p. 278)
6. myocardial infarction (p. 280)
7. HDL (p. 281)
8. chronic obstructive lung disease (p. 282)
9. lung (p. 283)
10. reduced (p. 284)

True or False

1. T (p. 284)
2. F (p. 284)
3. F (p. 285)
4. F (p. 285)
5. F (p. 285)
6. T (p. 286)
7. T (p. 286)
8. T (p. 289)
9. F (p. 290)
10. T (p. 274)

Multiple Choice

1. a (p. 274)
2. c (p. 274)
3. d (p. 274)
4. d (p. 276)
5. c (p. 277)
6. a (p. 286)
7. d (p. 282)
8. c (p. 282)
9. b (p. 284)
10. b (p. 285)

Turn to the back of the Study Guide, and complete Wellness Worksheets 42–45.

Chapter 12
Nutrition Basics

LEARNING OBJECTIVES

As a result of reading Chapter 12 in the textbook and completing the activities in this Study Guide, you should be able to do the following:

1. List the essential nutrients, and describe the functions they perform in the body.

2. Describe the Recommended Dietary Allowances, Food Guide Pyramid, and Dietary Guidelines for Americans.

3. Discuss nutritional guidelines for vegetarians and for special population groups.

4. Explain how to use food labels to make informed choices about foods.

5. Put together a personal nutrition plan based on affordable foods that you enjoy and that will promote wellness both now and in the future.

TERMINOLOGY

You should be able to define the following key terms:

amino acids
anemia
antioxidant
calcium
calorie
carbohydrate
certified organic
cholesterol
complete protein sources
complex carbohydrates
cruciferous vegetables
Daily Reference Values (DRV)
Daily Values
diabetes mellitus
Dietary Guidelines for Americans
dietary fiber
digestion
digestive enzymes
diverticulitis
enriched
essential amino acids
essential nutrients
fat-soluble vitamins
fats (lipids)

fatty acids
fish oils
Food Guide Pyramid
food irradiation
fortified
free radical
gallbladder disease
glucose
glycerol
glycogen
high-density lipoprotein (HDL)
hydrogenation
incomplete protein sources
insoluble fiber
iron
irritable bowel syndrome
kilocalorie
lacto-ovo-vegetarian
lacto-vegetarian
legumes
low-density lipoprotein (LDL)
metabolism
minerals
monosodium glutamate (MSG)

monounsaturated fat
nitrates
nitrites
nutrition
nutrition label
oat bran
oils
omega-3 fatty acid
omega-6 fatty acid
osteoporosis
partial, semivegetarian, or
    pescovegetarian
pathogen
peptic ulcers
phytochemical
polychlorinated biphenyl (PCB)
polyunsaturated fat
protein
psyllium
Recommended Dietary Allowances (RDAs)

Reference Daily Intakes (RDI)
registered dietitian
Salmonella poisoning
saturated fat
serum (blood) cholesterol
simple carbohydrates
soluble fiber
sulfites
supplements
tofu
trace minerals
trans fatty acid
scurvy
variety
vegan
vegetarian
vitamin deficiency diseases
vitamins
water-soluble vitamins

MAJOR POINTS AND ISSUES

1. Your nutritional lifestyle is an important determinant of your overall health. The average person spends, cumulatively, more than six years of life eating, and decisions that people make about the kinds and volume of food they eat contribute significantly to a person's overall wellness.

2. The average daily caloric need is about 2000 calories. The types of food that people eat vary substantially in their caloric density. Fats contain 9 calories per gram; alcohol, 7 calories per gram; proteins and carbohydrates, 4 calories per gram.

3. Proteins form the substantive parts of the body—bones and muscles. Most Americans consume more protein than they need, and because protein-rich foods are often high in fat, they also contribute to too much fat in the diet.

4. Fats are essential in the diet, but almost all Americans eat too much fat, some far in excess of their basic requirements, especially saturated fats.

5. Carbohydrates supply energy to the brain and other parts of the nervous system as well as red blood cells. Americans need to increase their consumption of complex carbohydrates and decrease the amount of simple carbohydrates consumed.

6. Dietary fiber includes plant substances difficult or impossible for humans to digest. Fiber may prevent colon cancer and help lower cholesterol levels. Fibers are classified as soluble and insoluble.

7. Vitamins are organic substances required in very small amounts to promote specific chemical reactions within living cells. A substance is considered a vitamin only if a lack of it causes a specific disease that is cured when the substance is resupplied. Humans need 13 vitamins.

8. Water is used to digest food, transport substances around the body, lubricate joints and organs, and regulate body temperature. Lack of water can cause death within a few days.

9. The 17 minerals needed in the diet are inorganic substances that regulate body functions, aid in growth and maintenance of body tissues, and act as catalysts for release of energy. Minerals most commonly lacking in the diet are iron, calcium, and zinc.

10. Recommended Daily Allowances (RDAs) are recommended intakes for essential nutrients that meet the needs of healthy persons. They are a guide to foods, not to supplements, and are averages for groups.

11. The Food Guide Pyramid translates nutrient recommendations into food group plans that ensure balanced intake of essential nutrients.

12. The Dietary Guidelines for Americans address prevention of diet-related diseases. The guidelines advise a person to eat a variety of foods, maintain desirable weight, avoid too much fat, eat adequate starch and fiber, avoid too much sugar, avoid too much sodium, and drink alcohol in moderation, if at all.

13. Aerobic exercises generate significant "free radicals;" consumption of antioxidants to offset those free radicals is recommended.

14. A vegetarian diet can meet human nutritional needs.

15. No single diet plan provides wellness for everyone.

16. Food labels provide ingredients in descending order based on weight. Almost all labels show how much fat, cholesterol, protein, fiber, and sodium foods contain. Serving sizes are standardized, and health claims are carefully regulated.

17. Most people don't need vitamin and mineral supplements, although pregnant and breastfeeding mothers and vegetarians are sometimes advised to use them.

18. Reliable nutritional advice can be obtained from registered dietitians.

19. The greatest threat to the safety of the food supply comes from bacteria and other microorganisms that cause foodborne illnesses.

20. Food additives are used to maintain or improve nutritional quality, maintain freshness, help in processing, and alter taste and appearance. Although concern about food additives is appropriate, suffering negative health consequences as a result of food additives is unlikely when a variety of foods are consumed in moderation.

21. Different populations have varied nutritional needs. Men often consume too many calories, teens too few. College students depend too heavily on fast food, and older people have declining nutritional needs. Athletes, especially, need to be sensitive to getting enough fluid.

SAMPLE TEST QUESTIONS

Completion

1. The energy in food is expressed as _____.

2. The food component that forms the muscles and bones is _____.

3. The food component with a caloric density of 9 calories per gram is _____.

4. The type of fat that most people should reduce most in their diet is _____ fat.

5. The food component that provides most energy during vigorous exercise is _____.

6. Instead of using laxatives, a person suffering from constipation may want to consume more _____ fiber to facilitate elimination.

7. The minerals most commonly lacking from the diet are _____, _____, and _____.

8. To compensate for the production of free radicals, people may want to increase consumption of fruits and vegetables, which are high in _____.

9. Some people who are concerned about the use of pesticides choose to buy foods that are certified _____.

10. The special population group that most needs to be conscious of remaining fully hydrated is _____.

True or False

1. The caloric density of alcohol is 7 calories per gram.

2. Hydrogenation is a process that makes fats healthy for consumption.

3. When unsaturated oils are hydrogenated, some trans fatty acids are produced.

4. The primary source of energy during athletic competition is fats.

5. A primary function of vitamins is to act as catalysts to initiate or speed up chemical reactions.

6. Vitamins C and E are antioxidant vitamins.

7. People who are most likely to need nutritional supplements include women with a heavy menstrual flow.

8. Most foodborne illness is due to *Staphylococcus aureua*.

9. Botulism is common and deadly.

10. "Certified organic" foods meet no additional standards and receive this designation based only on the whim of food producers.

Multiple Choice

1. The average daily caloric need for adults is approximately _____.
   a. 1200
   b. 1500
   c. 2000
   d. 2500

2. Proteins are divided into these categories:
   a. complete and incomplete
   b. complete and soluble
   c. incomplete and soluble
   d. complete and insoluble

3. The average American would benefit from this change in his or her diet:
   a. increasing simple carbohydrate intake
   b. increasing protein intake
   c. increasing consumption of vitamin supplements
   d. increasing intake of dietary fiber

4. To control cholesterol levels, the MOST important dietary step a person can take is:
   a. reduce simple carbohydrates
   b. reduce saturated fat
   c. reduce insoluble fiber
   d. reduce alcohol consumption

5. The best source of omega-3 fatty acids is a serving of:
   a. chicken breast
   b. pork chops
   c. salmon
   d. meat loaf

6. A recommended change in diet that makes sense is:
   a. increase carbohydrates and fats
   b. decrease carbohydrates and fats
   c. increase fats and reduce carbohydrates
   d. increase carbohydrates and reduce fats

7. What is the healthiest range for daily fiber consumption?
   a. 0-16 grams
   b. 16-20 grams
   c. 20-40 grams
   d. 60-80 grams

8. The American diet should often include more of the following EXCEPT:
   a. iron
   b. lead
   c. calcium
   d. zinc

9. Free radicals are increased as a result of:
   a. exposure to exhaust fumes
   b. consumption of too much fruit and fruit drinks
   c. limited exercise
   d. all of the above

10. Which of the following groups of foods should be consumed in the largest number of servings each day?
    a. bread, cereals, rice, pasta
    b. vegetables
    c. fruit
    d. milk, yogurt, cheese

SAMPLE TEST QUESTIONS ANSWER KEY

Completion

1. kilocalories (p. 300)
2. protein (p. 300)
3. fat (p. 301)
4. saturated (p. 302)
5. carbohydrates (p. 304)
6. insoluble (p. 308)
7. iron, calcium, zinc (p. 311)
8. antioxidants (p. 313)
9. organic (p. 330)
10. athletes (p. 323)

True or False

1. T (p. 300)
2. F (p. 302)
3. T (p. 303)
4. F (p. 304)
5. T (p. 308)
6. T (p. 310)
7. T (p. 325)
8. F (p. 329)
9. F (p. 329)
10. F (p. 330)

Multiple Choice

1. c (p. 300)
2. a (p. 300)
3. d (p. 308)
4. b (p. 303)
5. c (p. 304)
6. d (p. 307)
7. c (p. 308)
8. b (p. 311)
9. a (p. 313)
10. a (pp. 316–317)

Turn to the back of the Study Guide, and complete Wellness Worksheets 46–50.

Chapter 13
Exercise for Health and Fitness

LEARNING OBJECTIVES

As a result of reading Chapter 13 in the textbook and completing the activities in this Study Guide, you should be able to do the following:

1. Define physical fitness, and list the health-related components of fitness.

2. Explain the wellness benefits of exercise.

3. Describe how to develop each of the health-related components of fitness.

4. Discuss how to choose appropriate exercise equipment.

5. Describe eating and fluid consumption patterns a person should adopt to support regular vigorous exercise.

6. Describe how to assess fitness.

7. Discuss strategies for the prevention and treatment of exercise-induced injuries.

8. Create a personal exercise program that will facilitate the achievement of fitness goals.

TERMINOLOGY

You should be able to define the following key terms:

aerobic exercise
anabolic effects
anabolic steroids
body composition
cardiorespiratory endurance
cardiorespiratory endurance exercise
cardiovascular disease (CVD)
cool down
coronary heart disease
cross-training
dehydration
diabetes
duration
electrocardiogram (ECG or EKG)
endorphins
epinephrine

exercise
flexibility
frequency
high blood pressure
high-density lipoprotein (HDL)
intensity
isokinetic exercise
isometric exercise
isotonic exercise
lipids
lipoproteins
low-density lipoprotein (LDL)
maximal oxygen consumption (MOC)
medical clearance
metabolic rate
metabolism

muscular endurance

muscular strength

neurotransmitters

norepinephrine

osteoporosis

overload

physical fitness

physical training

resistive exercise

RICE principle

sedentary

skill training

stroke

synovial fluid

target heart rate

warm up

MAJOR POINTS AND ISSUES

1. The benefits of physical activity are varied. Benefits extend beyond physical activity to include mental well-being and are both short and long term. Regular physical activity is beneficial to almost everyone.

2. The five components most important to defining physical fitness are cardio-respiratory endurance, muscular strength, muscular endurance, flexibility, and body composition.

3. Specific benefits of regular exercise includes improved energy levels, enhanced emotional and psychological well-being, reduced risk of disease, reduced risk of injury and low-back pain, and reduced risk of premature death.

4. Regular physical activity improves body composition several ways, including increased calorie consumption, increased lean body mass, and increased metabolism.

5. The body works best when it is active. Left unchallenged, bones lose their density, joints stiffen, muscles become weak, and body chemistry and systems begin to degenerate. To truly be well, you must be active.

6. Criteria for designing your own fitness plan include age, frequency, intensity, and duration of exercise session.

7. Walking, if done briskly enough and long enough, can be effective in achieving a high level of fitness.

8. Activities best for achieving cardiorespiratory endurance are walking, jogging, running, swimming, bicycling, and aerobic exercise.

9. The primary purpose of endurance training is to increase maximal oxygen consumption.

10. Warm-up and cool-down exercises prepare the body for exercise and reduce the likelihood of injuries.

11. Three types of strength training exercises are resistive, isotonic, and isometric.

12. A primary advantage of weight machines versus free weights is safety. Free weights require more care, balance, and coordination to use.

13. Strength training exercises cause somewhat different changes in men and women. In men, muscles become larger and stronger, and in women, strength is increased and body fat is lost.

14. Stretching is an important, albeit often neglected, part of a fitness program.

15. Keeping satisfactorily hydrated is important during exercise. Drink frequently during exercise, and do not rely on thirst to determine when to consume fluids.

16. There are four basic steps to rehabilitation after an injury. Reduce the level of inflammation using the RICE (Rest, Ice, Compression, Elevation) principle; gradually exercise to restore normal joint motion, normal strength and endurance, and functional capacity.

SAMPLE TEST QUESTIONS

Completion

1. The total percentage of Americans who are completely sedentary or not regularly active is _____.

2. The body's ability to perform prolonged, large-muscle exercise at a moderate to high level is termed _____.

3. A physically fit person does muscle development exercise for _____ and _____.

4. The proportion of fat to lean tissue is termed _____.

5. The four major risk factors for cardiovascular disease include smoking, high cholesterol levels, high blood pressure, and _____ .

6. Moderate endurance exercise helps the immune system to function _____.

7. The first step in initiating an exercise program for a person who has been inactive for years is to get _____.

8. The amount of overload needed for a particular level of fitness is determined in terms of frequency, duration, and _____.

9. As a rule of thumb, you should drink about 8 ounces of water for every _____ minutes of heavy exercise.

10. Athletic injuries should be treated using the R-I-C-E principle of rest, ice, _____, and elevation.

True or False

1. To continue to improve physical fitness, you should progressively increase your exercise overload.

2. Regardless of the type of exercise, optimal development will occur when exercising three times per week.

3. Optimal physical development for recreational athletes occurs when aerobic activities are performed 5 to 7 days per week.

4. Stretching exercises will result in the most flexibility if done after exercise.

5. A primary purpose of endurance training is to increase maximal oxygen consumption.

6. Physical fitness will increase fastest after the sixth month of physical training.

7. During exercise half of the blood volume is directed to the muscles.

8. Strength training using weight machines develops strength more adaptable to everyday life than strength training using free weights.

9. Using steroids may cause a male's testes to atrophy.

10. After the swelling from an athletic injury has subsided, heat can be applied to speed up the healing process.

Multiple Choice

1. The percentage of Americans who do not exercise at all is:
   a. 25%
   b. 40%
   c. 65%
   d. 80%

2. The element of fitness that requires the MOST frequent exercise to maintain is:
   a. cardiorespiratory endurance
   b. muscular strength
   c. flexibility
   d. speed

3. Body composition refers to the relative amounts of _____ in a person's body or life.
   a. exercise and body fat
   b. exercise and lean tissue
   c. frequency of exercise and intensity of exercise
   d. body fat and lean tissue

4. The blood fats that increase with exercise are:
   a. very-low-density lipoproteins
   b. low-density lipoproteins
   c. high-density lipoproteins
   d. triglycerides

5. Regular exercisers are at lower risk for:
   a. stroke
   b. cancer
   c. Type 2 diabetes
   d. all of the above

6. Which of the following exercises does NOT protect women against osteoporosis?
   a. jogging
   b. aerobic dance
   c. swimming
   d. stair climbing

7. Exercise intensity is measured by:
   a. a clock
   b. pulse rate
   c. check list
   d. number of exercise sessions per week

8. Optimal cardiovascular endurance will occur with _____ exercise sessions per week.
   a. 2
   b. 3
   c. 4
   d. 5

9. The training effect is best achieved by exercise at _____% of maximal heart rate.
   a. 20–25
   b. 40–70
   c. 60–90
   d. 75–100

10. Warm-up exercises
    a. help spread synovial fluid
    b. tighten muscles
    c. strengthen muscles
    d. equalize blood flow

SAMPLE TEST QUESTIONS ANSWER KEY

Completion

1. 85% (p. 338)
2. cardiorespiratory endurance (p. 338)
3. strength, endurance (p. 339)
4. body composition (p. 340)
5. inactivity (pp. 341–342)
6. better (p. 344)
7. medical clearance (p. 348)
8. intensity (p. 346)
9. 30 (p. 360)
10. compression (p. 361)

True or False

1. T (p. 346)
2. F (p. 346)
3. F (p. 346)
4. T (p. 353)
5. T (p. 349)
6. F (p. 349)
7. F (p. 350)
8. F (p. 351)
9. T (p. 353)
10. T (p. 361)

Multiple Choice

1. a (p. 338)
2. b (p. 346)
3. d (p. 341)
4. c (p. 342)
5. d (p. 342)
6. c (p. 342)
7. b (p. 348)
8. d (p. 348)
9. c (p. 349)
10. a (p. 350)

Turn to the back of the Study Guide, and complete Wellness Worksheets 51–54.

Chapter 14
Weight Management

LEARNING OBJECTIVES

As a result of reading Chapter 14 in the textbook and completing the activities in this Study Guide, you should be able to do the following:

1. Explain the health risks associated with obesity.

2. Discuss different methods for assessing body weight and body composition.

3. Explain factors that may contribute to a weight problem, including genetic, environmental, and personal considerations.

4. Describe lifestyle factors that contribute to weight gain and loss, including the roles of diet, exercise, and emotional factors.

5. Identify and describe the symptoms of eating disorders and the health risks associated with them.

6. Design a personal plan for successfully managing body weight.

TERMINOLOGY

You should be able to define the following key terms:

adipose tissue
amenorrhea
anorexia nervosa
binge-eating disorder
binge-purge cycle
blood sugar level
body composition
body image
body mass index (BMI)
bulimia nervosa
calipers
calories
complex carbohydrates
dexfenfluramine
dietary supplements
eating disorders
electrical impedance analysis
energy balance
essential fat

fat
fenfluramine
fiber
gastroplasty
genetic factors
height-weight charts
hunger
hydrostatic weighing
lean body mass
leptin
liposuction
metabolism
nonessential (storage) fat
obesity
overfat
overweight
percent body fat
phentermine
phenylpropanolamine hydrochloride

protein
purging
resting metabolic rate (RMR)
satiety
scanning procedures
severe obesity

simple carbohydrates
simple sugars
skinfold measurement
underwater weighing
very-low-calorie diet (VLCD)
weight cycling

MAJOR POINTS AND ISSUES

1. Being overfat is a significant health risk for many individuals and a serious public health challenge for the United States.

2. Among Americans, both the prevalence of obesity and the number of people who are dieting is continuing to rise.

3. The human body is divided into lean body mass and fat tissue. Lean body mass includes all of the body's nonfat tissues (bone, water, muscle, connective tissues and organs, and teeth).

4. Overconsumption of dietary fat is a major problem in the American diet.

5. The most important consideration in looking at body weight is the percent of body fat.

6. The key to keeping a healthy ratio of fat to lean body mass is maintaining a balance between energy (calories) consumed and expended.

7. There are significant health risks associated with being too fat. They include increased risk of hypertension, diabetes, some types of cancer, impaired immune function, gallbladder and kidney diseases, and impaired psychological health.

8. Although the majority of weight-related health problems result from too much fat, some people are too lean. Among women, being excessively lean is associated with amenorrhea and loss of bone mass.

9. A variety of techniques are used to accurately assess body composition. They include hydrostatic weighing, skinfold measurements, electrical impedance analysis, and scanning procedures. Height-weight charts are a less accurate basis on which to judge one's need to lose weight.

10. Multiple factors determine if a person has a weight problem. Genetics influences body size and shape, body fat distribution, and metabolic rate. Exercise and eating patterns are also very important determinants of body weight.

11. Physical, psychological, social, and cultural factors can all play a role in weight problems.

12. Maintaining a healthy weight for a lifetime is not the product of dieting. Lifestyle factors are critical for successful long-term weight management.

13. Energy balance describes the practice of consuming a number of calories approximately equal to the amount of calories expended in daily activities.

14. Successful weight management is assisted by limiting dietary fat to no more than 30% of total calories, increasing the consumption of complex carbohydrates, and eating small, frequent meals.

15. Regular physical activity is critical to successful weight management. It is recommended that all Americans accumulate 30 minutes or more of moderate-intensity physical activity on most days.

16. For people who are more than 20% overweight, consideration of more drastic weight-management measures may be appropriate, including prescription medications and surgery.

17. Although less than 3% of Americans suffer from eating disorders, they are serious threats to health and, for some people, ultimately result in premature death.

SAMPLE TEST QUESTIONS

Completion

1. The two components of body composition are _____ and _____.

2. Obesity is usually defined as _____% or more overweight.

3. A person's mental picture of her/his own body is defined as _____.

4. Calipers are used to make _____ measurements to determine body composition.

5. Underwater weighing is one of the most accurate means of assessing body composition and is also known as _____ weighing.

6. The largest component in metabolism is the _____.

7. The element of the diet that should make up 55–60% of all calories consumed is _____.

8. Fat calories should make up a maximum of _____% of all calories consumed.

9. Anorexia nervosa typically develops in girls between the ages of _____ and _____.

10. Compulsive overeaters generally eat as a result of stress or other emotions, not as a result of _____.

True or False

1. Dietary protein should make up about 40% of the daily diet.

2. To lose weight, it's best to declare some foods permanently "off limits."

3. The recommended amount of physical activity on most days is 15 minutes.

4. Genetic factors have been rejected as contributors to body weight.

5. An important component of a weight-loss program is a balanced diet.

6. The most common ingredient in diet aids is phenylpropanolamine hydrochloride (PPA).

7. The level of obesity that indicates a medically supervised very-low-calorie diet is 100% or more overweight.

8. More people suffer from anorexia than from bulimia.

9. Included among the health consequences of anorexia nervosa is limited tolerance for cold.

10. Low income appears to be related to being overweight.

Multiple Choice

1. Which of the following is probably MOST responsible for lack of success in weight management?
   a. eating too many carbohydrates
   b. eating too little fat
   c. eating too much protein
   d. concentrating on short-term weight loss

2. Lean body mass includes all of the following EXCEPT:
   a. fat
   b. bone
   c. muscle
   d. connective issue

3. Body types are sometimes described as being like different fruits. Which of the following body type labels is MOST closely associated with elevated risk of heart disease, high blood pressure, and stroke:
   a. pear
   b. apple
   c. berry
   d. banana

4. Body image is determined by:
    a. one's own thinking
    b. hydrostatic weighing
    c. height-weight charts
    d. calculation of body mass index

5. The LEAST accurate means of determining if a person is too fat is:
    a. hydrostatic weighing
    b. electrical impedance analysis
    c. skin caliper measurements
    d. height-weight charts

6. The fat cell theory suggests that fat stored in the body results from:
    a. too little exercise
    b. too much food consumption
    c. the number and size of fat cells in the body
    d. genetics

7. The greatest portion of the diet should be made up of _____.
    a. fat
    b. sugar
    c. protein
    d. carbohydrates

8. The contemporary recommendation for exercise is a minimum of
_____ minutes of moderate-intensity physical activity most days.
    a. 10
    b. 15
    c. 20
    d. 30

9. Stomach stapling is also called:
    a. gastric resectioning
    b. gastroplasty
    c. liposuction
    d. none of the above

10. A factor involved in the development of an eating disorder is:
    a. insensitivity to others
    b. stable family environment
    c. low socioeconomic status
    d. dissatisfaction with body image

SAMPLE TEST QUESTIONS ANSWER KEY

Completion

1. lean body mass, body fat (p. 370)
2. 20 (p. 371)
3. body image (p. 372)
4. skinfold (p. 374)
5. hydrostatic (p. 374)
6. resting metabolic rate (p. 377)
7. carbohydrates (p. 382)
8. 30 (p. 380)
9. 12, 18 (p. 389)
10. hunger (p. 391)

True or False

1. F (p. 382)
2. F (p. 382)
3. F (p. 382)
4. F (pp. 381–382)
5. T (pp. 380–382)
6. T (p. 386)
7. T (p. 388)
8. F (p. 389)
9. T (p. 390)
10. T (p. 371)

Multiple Choice

1. d (p. 370)
2. a (p. 370)
3. b (pp. 371–372)
4. a (p. 372)
5. d (p. 374)
6. c (p. 377)
7. d (p. 382)
8. d (p. 382)
9. b (p. 389)
10. d (p. 387)

Turn to the back of the Study Guide, and complete Wellness Worksheets 55–59.

Chapter 15
Cardiovascular Health

LEARNING OBJECTIVES

As a result of reading Chapter 15 in the textbook and completing the activities in this Study Guide, you should be able to do the following:

1. List the major components of the cardiovascular system.

2. Describe how blood is pumped and circulated throughout the body.

3. Describe the controllable and uncontrollable risk factors associated with cardiovascular disease.

4. Discuss the major forms of cardiovascular disease and how they develop.

5. List steps that you can take to lower your personal risk of developing cardiovascular disease.

TERMINOLOGY

You should be able to define the following key terms:

aneurysm
angina pectoris
angiogram (arteriogram)
aorta
arrhythmia
arteries
arteriogram
arterioles
arteriosclerosis
atherosclerosis
atria
balloon angioplasty
beta-blockers
blood cholesterol
blood pressure
capillaries
carbon dioxide
cardiopulmonary resuscitation (CPR)
cardiovascular disease (CVD)
cardiovascular system
carotid artery
cerebral artery

cerebral embolism
cerebral hemorrhage
cerebral thrombosis
Chlamydia pneumoniae
cholesterol
coarctation of the aorta
collateral circulation
computed tomography (CT)
congenital heart disease
congestive heart failure
coronary arteries
coronary bypass surgery
coronary heart disease (CHD)
coronary occlusion
coronary thrombosis
cutaneous transluminal angioplasty
cytomegalovirus
defibrillator
diabetes
diastole
dietary cholesterol
diuretics

electrocardiogram (ECG or EKG)
electroencephalogram (EEG)
embolus
essential hypertension
heart attack
helicobacter pylori
high-density lipoprotein (HDL)
homocysteine
hypertension
low-density lipoprotein (LDL)
lung surfactant
magnetic resonance imaging (MRI)
monounsaturated fat
myocardial infarction
obesity
oxygen
pacemaker
plaque
platelets
polyunsaturated fat
pulmonary artery
pulmonary circulation
pulmonary edema
radionuclide imaging

rheumatic fever
rheumatic heart disease
risk factors
saturated fats
secondary hypertension
sedentary lifestyle
sphygmomanometer
stroke
systemic circulation
systole
thrombus
total cholesterol
transient ischemic attack (TIA)
triglycerides
Type A personality
Type B personality
Type D personality
vasodilators
veins
vena cava
ventricles
venules
very-low-density lipoprotein (VLDL)

MAJOR POINTS/ISSUES

1. Cardiovascular disease is the number one killer in the United States. Almost half of all people alive today will die from heart disease.

2. The cardiovascular system, which consists of the heart and blood vessels, pumps and circulates blood throughout the body; the pulmonary and systemic circulation systems are controlled by the right and left sides of the heart, respectively.

3. The heart is a four-chambered organ about the size of a fist. The atria are the thin-walled upper chambers, and the ventricles are the thick-walled lower chambers.

4. The heart beats when ventricles contract (systole), pumping blood to the lungs via the pulmonary artery and to the body via the aorta and the entire arterial system. When the heart relaxes between beats (diastole), blood flows from the atria into the ventricles.

5. The total volume of the body's blood, about 5 quarts in a 150-pound man, circulates in about one minute, with exchange of nutrients taking place between the capillaries and the tissues.

6. Major risk factors for CVD that can be changed are tobacco use, high blood pressure, unhealthy cholesterol levels, and a sedentary lifestyle.

8. The risk of CVD increases as blood cholesterol increases. The National Cholesterol Education Program (NCEP) recommends testing at least once every five years for all adults, beginning at age 20.

9. Cholesterol levels can be changed through diet, exercise, smoking cessation, and medication.

10. Contributing risk factors for CVD that can be changed include overweight, diabetes, stress, a chronically hostile personality, and lack of social support.

11. Major risk factors for CVD that cannot be changed are heredity, aging, being male, and certain factors associated with race or ethnicity.

12. Atherosclerosis is the process whereby arteries become narrowed by deposits of fat, cholesterol, and other substances. Results of this process include hypertension, heart attack, angina pectoris, and stroke.

13. An estimated 60 million Americans have high blood pressure, often called the "silent killer" because there are usually no symptoms, even as damage to vital organs is occurring. High blood pressure in adults is defined as systolic pressure of 140 mm Hg or higher and diastolic pressure of 90 mm Hg or higher.

14. Potential cardiovascular disease factors currently the focus of considerable research are: triglycerides, homocysteine, lipoprotein(a), and some infectious agents.

15. Hypertension, depending on its type and severity, can be treated by restricting salt intake, losing weight, and/or through the use of antihypertensive drugs.

16. Heart attacks and strokes are usually the end result of a long disease process. It is important to recognize the signals of a heart attack so that the victim can be transported to an emergency facility. Immediate care, often essential for survival, includes cardiopulmonary resuscitation, defibrillation, and administration of "clot-busting" drugs.

17. Heart disease can be diagnosed through the use of stress or exercise tests. Magnetic resonance imaging, nuclear magnetic resonance imaging, and radionuclide imaging are methods of assessing the heart disease patient's condition. Treatments for heart disease include balloon angioplasty, percutaneous transluminal angioplasty, and coronary bypass surgery.

18. The three major types of strokes are thrombotic strokes, embolic strokes, and hemorrhagic strokes. Strokes usually lead to some lasting disability. Effective treatment depends in part on prompt recognition of symptoms and correct diagnosis of the type of stroke.

19. Congestive heart failure results if the heart is weakened and is unable to pump out all the blood that returns to it. Fluid can collect in the lungs and interfere with breathing.

20. People need to take steps beginning when they are young to improve chances of avoiding CVD in middle age. These steps include having blood pressure checked regularly, monitoring blood cholesterol, quitting smoking, eating a healthy diet, maintaining an ideal weight, exercising regularly, managing stress effectively, controlling medical problems, developing effective ways to deal with anger, and knowing your own CVD risk factors, both personal and familial.

96

SAMPLE TEST QUESTIONS

Completion

1. The leading cause of death in the United States is _____.

2. The blood vessels that branch off the aorta and carry blood back to the heart are the _____.

3. The "good" cholesterol is _____.

4. The "bad" cholesterol is _____.

5. The most important behavior related to prevention of cardiovascular disease is _____.

6. The elements of the Type A personality that are associated with increased risk of heart attack are _____, _____, and _____.

7. The personality that is characterized by pessimism, negativity, and suppression of negative feelings is a _____ personality.

8. A heart attack caused by a clot is called a _____.

9. When the heart cannot pump adequately and fluids back up in the body, the process is known as _____.

10. Changing to a heart-healthy diet involves cutting fat intake, substituting unsaturated for saturated fats, and increasing intake of _____.

True or False

1. Death rates from heart disease are almost identical among ethnic groups in the United States.

2. Angina pain is an early warning that the load on the heart must be reduced.

3. Most congenital heart disease can be treated with medication or surgery.

4. The National Cholesterol Education Program recommends that everyone over the age of 55 limit fat consumption to 30% of all calories.

5. It is recommended that everyone consume 20–35 grams of dietary fiber daily.

6. Excessive salt consumption is equally risky for all Americans.

7. A person who once smoked and quit always has a greater risk of CVD than a person who never smoked.

8. Almost all hypertensive Americans have their blood pressure under control.

9. Total cholesterol levels in excess of 180 indicate a need for therapeutic intervention.

10. Small doses of aspirin may benefit people at elevated risk for cardiovascular disease by reducing the tendency of blood to clot.

Multiple Choice

1. After the blood leaves the left ventricle it goes to the:
    a. left atrium
    b. lungs
    c. right ventricle
    d. rest of the body

2. After the blood leaves the right atrium it goes to the:
    a. right ventricle
    b. left atrium
    c. brain
    d. lungs

3. Blood goes into the coronary artery from the:
    a. heart
    b. aorta
    c. superior vena cava
    d. inferior vena cava

4. The element in blood that reduces the risk of heart disease is:
    a. high-density lipoprotein
    b. low-density lipoprotein
    c. very-low-density lipoprotein
    d. triglycerides

5. "Bad" cholesterol is also labeled:
    a. high-density lipoprotein
    b. low-density lipoprotein
    c. homocysteine
    d. lipoprotein(a)

6. Dietary changes that can protect against cardiovascular disease include all of the following EXCEPT:
    a. decreasing fiber intake
    b. decreasing fat intake
    c. replacing animal proteins with soy proteins
    d. increasing fish and seafood consumption

7. All of the following elements of Type A personalities put a person at elevated risk for heart disease EXCEPT:
    a. time sensitivity
    b. anger
    c. hostility
    d. cynicism

8. Which of the following is NOT a characteristic of the Type D personality?
   a. pessimism
   b. negativity
   c. suppression of negative feelings
   d. eagerness

9. The age at which heart attack risk increases dramatically is:
   a. 45
   b. 55
   c. 65
   d. 75

10. The infectious agent that is the focus of current research as a cause of heart disease is:
    a. HIV
    b. cytomegalovirus
    c. chlamydia
    d. lipoprotein(a)

SAMPLE TEST QUESTIONS ANSWER KEY

Completion

1. cardiovascular disease (p. 398)
2. coronary arteries (p. 399)
3. high-density lipoproteins (p. 400)
4. low-density lipoproteins (p. 401)
5. physical activity (p. 403)
6. hostility, cynicism, anger (p. 404)
7. Type D (p. 404)
8. coronary thrombosis (p. 411)
9. congestive heart failure (p. 415)
10. fiber (p. 416)

True or False

1. F (p. 406)
2. T (p. 411)
3. T (p. 416)
4. F (p. 416)
5. T (p. 416)
6. F (p. 417)
7. F (p. 419)
8. F (p. 419)
9. F (p. 419)
10. T (p. 419)

Multiple Choice

1. d (p. 398)
2. a (p. 398)
3. b (p. 398)
4. a (p. 401)
5. b (p. 401)
6. a (pp. 416–417)
7. a (p. 404)
8. d (p. 404)
9. c (p. 405)
10. b (p. 408)

Turn to the back of the Study Guide, and complete Wellness Worksheets 60–63.

Chapter 16
Cancer

LEARNING OBJECTIVES

As a result of reading Chapter 16 in the textbook and completing the activities in this Study Guide, you should be able to do the following:

1. Explain what cancer is and how it spreads.

2. List and describe common cancers.

3. Identify common risk factors for cancer.

4. Identify the common signs and symptoms of cancer.

5. Discuss customary cancer treatments.

6. Describe successful strategies for cancer prevention.

7. Discuss some of the causes of cancer and how they can be minimized or prevented.

8. Describe common cancer screening procedures.

9. Describe approaches to making definitive cancer diagnoses.

10. List specific actions you can take to lower your risk of cancer.

TERMINOLOGY

You should be able to define the following key terms:

anticarcinogen
antioxidant
basal cell carcinoma
benign
benign tumor
biological therapies
biopsy
bladder cancer
bone marrow
bone marrow transplantation
brachytherapy
breast cancer
breast self-examination
cancer
cancer promoter
carcinogen

carcinoma
carotenoid
cervical cancer
chemotherapy
chromosomes
colon and rectal cancer
computerized tomography(CT)
cytokine
DNA
diethylstilbestrol (DES)
endometrial cancer
endometrium
epithelial layer
free radicals
gene
genetic susceptibility

Hodgkin's disease
immune system
immunotherapy
impotence
incontinence
induction chemo-therapy
Kaposi's sarcoma
leukemia
lumpectomy
lung cancer
lymph nodes
lymphatic circulation
lymphatic system
lymphoma
magnetic resonance imaging (MRI)
malignant
malignant neoplasm
malignant tumor
mammography
mastectomy
melanoma
metastasis
mutagen
nitrosamine
oncogene
oncologist
oral cancer
ovarian cancer
palpation
pancreatic cancer

Pap test
phytochemical
polyp
primary prevention
primary tumor
prognosis
prostate cancer
prostate-specific antigen (PSA)
protease inhibitor
PSA blood test
radiation
radiation therapy
remission
sarcoma
secondary prevention
secondary tumors (metastases)
sigmoidoscope
skin cancer
sputum
squamous cell carcinoma
sulforaphane
sunscreen
suppressor gene
surgery
survival rate
testicular cancer
tumor
ultrasonography
ultraviolet (UV) radiation

MAJOR POINTS/ISSUES

1. Cancer is an abnormal and uncontrollable growth of cells or tissue that leads to death if untreated. More than half of all cancers in the United States can be prevented.

2. A malignant tumor can invade surrounding structure and spread—metastasize—to distant sites via the blood and lymphatic system, producing additional tumors throughout the body.

3. Unlike normal cells, malignant cells divide at a much more rapid rate.

4. Malignant tumors are classified according to the types of cells that give rise to them. The most common cancers are carcinomas, sarcomas, lymphomas, and leukemia.

5. About one-third of all Americans will contract cancer. Of these, nearly 60% will be "cured."

6. Lung cancer is the most common cancer in the United States and is very difficult to detect at an early stage. Smoking is the primary cause of lung cancer.

7. Colorectal cancer, the second most common cause of cancer death in the United States, is clearly linked to both diet and heredity.

8. About 110 per 100,000 women in the United States develops breast cancer per year. Risk factors include heredity, hormonal factors, and lifestyle. The American Cancer Society recommends monthly self-examination for all women over 20, a clinical examination every three years, and regular mammograms after 40.

9. A new blood test measures the amount of prostate-specific antigen (PSA) in the blood and can be helpful in diagnosing prostate cancer. Early detection leads to a higher survival rate.

10. Prostate cancer is the most common cancer in men and is chiefly a disease of aging.

11. Cervical cancer is, at least in part, a sexually transmitted disease. Probably more than 80% of cervical cancer stems from infection with human papillomavirus, which is transmitted during unprotected sex.

12. Uterine cancer is diagnosed most often in women over the age of 55. Uterine cancer risk factors are similar to those for breast cancer.

13. Ovarian cancer is relatively rare, but more frequently fatal to those who contract it, because screening and diagnostic techniques do not usually identify it until it is too late for successful treatment.

14. The incidence of skin cancer has increased dramatically in recent years. Depletion of the ozone layer has been implicated in the increased incidence of skin cancer; using sunscreen for protection against ultraviolet rays continues to be of primary importance. Basal cell and squamous cell carcinomas are easily treatable; melanoma is much less common but much more deadly. The ABCD test can help detect melanoma.

15. Oral cancer is caused primarily by various forms of tobacco use.

16. Testicular cancer can be detected through self-examination.

17. Some behavioral choices may contribute to DNA copying errors that contribute to cancer risk. These include smoking and unprotected sex.

18. Some cancers have a genetic basis and risk can be inherited.

19. Different foods can contain cancer-preventing as well as cancer-causing compounds. Individuals can affect their cancer risk through dietary changes.

20. Carcinogens in the environment include food additives, pollution, and radiation. All sources of radiation are potentially carcinogenic.

21. Early detection of cancer is critical in terms of treatment and outcome. Self-monitoring, screening tests, and advanced technological developments have all made early detection possible for many types of cancer.

22. The American Cancer Society has identified seven warning signs of cancer: change in bowel or bladder habits, a sore that does not heal, unusual bleeding or discharge, thickening or lump in the breasts or elsewhere, indigestion or difficulty in swallowing, obvious change in a wart or mole, and nagging cough or hoarseness. Although none of these signs is a clear indication of cancer, any one of them should send you to your physician for further investigation.

23. Traditional cancer treatment methods consist of surgery, chemotherapy, and radiation therapy. Immunotherapy, vaccines, and genetic engineering also hold promise as effective treatments.

24. Primary prevention involves making choices to avoid cancer-causing substances in the environment. Secondary prevention involves early detection of cancers that do occur.

25. Lifestyle is a strong predictor of cancer risk. Studies show that an altered lifestyle can reduce the risk of cancer by as much as 50 percent.

SAMPLE TEST QUESTIONS

Completion

1. A tumor that is made up of cells that are similar to the surrounding normal cells and are enclosed in a membrane that prevents them from penetrating neighboring tissues is called a _____ tumor.

2. The process by which cancer cells spread through the body is _____ .

3. Breast cancer has been surpassed by _____ cancer as the major cause of death in women.

4. The type of cancer that is at least partly a sexually transmitted disease is _____ cancer.

5. Screening for changes in cervical cells that precede cancer is done primarily by means of a _____ test.

6. The female reproductive tract cancer that is most difficult to diagnose at a stage that permits successful intervention is _____ cancer.

7. The most dangerous form of skin cancer is _____.

8. Any change in the normal sequence of nucleotide bases in a gene is called a _____.

9. Substances in plants that help protect against chronic diseases such as cancer are _____.

10. The seven warning signs of cancer can be remembered using the acronym
_____.

True or False

1. Oral cancer is associated with both tobacco use and excessive use of alcohol.

2. Men are most likely to contract testicular cancer after age 40.

3. Bladder cancer is more common in women than men.

4. The chance of any American contracting cancer is her/his lifetime is 50%.

5. Diet is not a factor in the incidence of colon cancer.

6. Mammography for all women between the ages of 40 and 50 is universally recommended.

7. The strongest predictor of prostate cancer is age.

8. Almost all cases of skin cancer can be traced to excessive exposure to UV radiation.

9. The food we eat can increase our cancer risk, but there are no foods that reduce cancer risk.

10. Alcohol consumption is associated with several cancers, including an apparent link with breast cancer.

Multiple Choice

1. The percentage of all cancers that could be prevented by simple lifestyle changes is:
   a. 20%
   b. 30%
   c. 40%
   d. 50%

2. The least serious type of tumor is:
   a. cancerous
   b. benign
   c. malignant
   d. all of these types of tumors are life threatening

3. Cancer in the blood-forming cells is called:
   a. carcinoma
   b. sarcoma
   c. lymphoma
   d. leukemia

4. Cancer that arises from the epithelial layers is called:
   a. carcinoma
   b. sarcoma
   c. lymphoma
   d. leukemia

5. Cancer that attacks the body's infection-fighting system is called:
    a. carcinoma
    b. sarcoma
    c. lymphoma
    d. leukemia

6. Cancer that arises from connective and fibrous tissue is called:
    a. carcinoma
    b. sarcoma
    c. lymphoma
    d. leukemia

7. The most deadly form of female reproductive tract cancer is:
    a. cervical cancer
    b. uterine cancer
    c. endometrial cancer
    d. ovarian cancer

8. The most common form of cancer is:
    a. lung cancer
    b. breast cancer
    c. skin cancer
    d. prostate cancer

9. Breast cancer increases in women that drink:
    a. nonfat or skim milk
    b. phytochemically-enhanced juices
    c. any alcohol at all
    d. at least three alcoholic drinks per day

10. All of the following are associated with increased cancer risk EXCEPT:
    a. high-fiber diet
    b. high-fat diet
    c. high alcohol consumption
    d. exposure to smog

SAMPLE TEST QUESTIONS ANSWER KEY

Completion

1. benign (p. 428)
2. metastasis (p. 428)
3. lung (p. 430)
4. cervical (p. 434)
5. Pap (p. 434)
6. ovarian (p. 436)
7. melanoma (p. 438)
8. mutation (p. 442)
9. phytochemicals (p. 445)
10. CAUTION (p. 449)

True or False

1. T (p. 439)
2. F (p. 440)
3. F (p. 440)
4. F (p. 430)
5. F (p. 431)
6. F (p. 432)
7. T (p. 433)
8. T (p. 437)
9. F (p. 443)
10. T (p. 444)

Multiple Choice

1. d (p. 428)
2. b (p. 428)
3. d (p. 430)
4. a (p. 430)
5. c (p. 430)
6. b (p. 430)
7. d (p. 436)
8. c (p. 437)
9. d (p. 444)
10. a (p. 444)

Turn to the back of the Study Guide, and complete Wellness Worksheets 64–66.

Chapter 17
Immunity and Infection

LEARNING OBJECTIVES

As a result of reading Chapter 17 in the textbook and completing the activities in this Study Guide, you should be able to do the following:

1. Describe the step-by-step process by which infectious diseases are transmitted.

2. List the body's physical and chemical barriers to infection.

3. Explain how the immune system responds to an invading microorganism.

4. List the major types of pathogens.

5. Describe the most common diseases caused by pathogens.

6. Discuss steps you can take to prevent infections and strengthen your immune system.

TERMINOLOGY

You should be able to define the following key terms:

acquired immunity
active immunity
adaptive or acquired immunity
African sleeping sickness
allergen
allergy
amoebic dysentery
antibody
antibody-mediated immune response
antigen
anti-inflammatory medication
autoimmune disease
B cell
bacillus
bacterium
Candida albicans
cell-mediated immune response
chemical barriers
chlamydia
cilia

coccidioidomycosis
contagious
contagious disease
cytokine
enzyme
Epstein-Barr virus (EBV)
fever
flukes
fungus
gamma globulin
gram-negative bacteria
gram-positive bacteria
helper T cells
herpesvirus
histamine
histoplasmosis
HIV
host
immune response
immune system

immunity
immunization
incubation
infection
inflammatory response
influenza
ingestion
inhalation
interferon
interleukin
killer T cell
local infection
lymph nodes
lymphatic system
lymphocytes
macrophage
malaria
memory B cell
memory T cell
mycoplasma
natural killer cell
neutrophil
opportunistic infection
parasite
parasitic worm
passive immunity

pathogen
phagocytic cell
physical barriers
poliomyelitis
portal of entry
portal of exit
prodromal period
prodrome
protozoan
reservoir
rickettsia
routes of infection
spirochete
staphylococcus
streptococcus
stress
supressor T cell
systemic infection
T cell
tetanus
toxin
tuberculosis (TB)
vaccine
vector
virus

MAJOR POINTS AND ISSUES

1. The immune system works to protect the body from infectious agents from the outside and from changes on the inside, such as cancer.

2. The body has effective systems for protecting it against illness. These systems include the skin, mucous membranes, and antibody-rich fluids (tears, saliva, vaginal secretions).

3. The chain of infection has six major links: pathogen, reservoir, portal of exit, means of transmission, portal of entry, and new host.

4. There are multiple strategies to prevent the spread of infection, including development of public health policies and medical intervention. All these strategies are ultimately targeted at breaking the "chain of infection."

5. The immune system is an elaborate and complicated internal system that responds to foreign organisms once they have invaded the body. The immune response has four major phases: (1) recognition of the invading pathogen, (2) amplification of defenses, (3) attack, and (4) slowdown.

6. Many illnesses are unlikely to strike the same person twice due to elevated immunity that is produced by the first bout with the disease.

7. Immunity can be achieved without being sick. An antigen similar to the disease-causing organism is introduced into the body via a vaccination. Immunity develops as a result of this process without causing illness.

8. Allergies are an inappropriate response by the immune system. An allergic reaction is the body's immune system responding to a harmless substance such as airborne dust.

9. Disease-causing pathogens include bacteria, viruses, fungi, protozoa, and parasitic worms.

10. Aggressive treatment of bacterial infections has produced antibiotic-resistant bacteria. To counter the trend toward "tougher" bacteria you should not demand an antibiotic every time you are sick or take an antibiotic without a prescription, and you should always use antibiotics as directed when they are prescribed.

11. A variety of circumstances influences the effectiveness of our immune systems, including the amount of stress in our lives and up-to-date immunizations.

SAMPLE TEST QUESTIONS

Completion

1. The primary physical barrier to pathogens attempting to enter the body is the _____.

2. The last link in the chain of infection is the _____.

3. The natural environment in which a pathogen typically resides is called the _____.

4. Skin penetration, inhalation, and ingestion are all portals of _____ for pathogens.

5. T cells and B cells are types of _____.

6. The inflammatory response causes the blood vessels to dilate and fluid to flow out of the capillaries to the injured tissue. The bodily ingredient that causes this specific reaction is _____.

7. The first phase of the immune response is the _____.

8. After a person recovers from an illness, _____ protects him or her from a similar future illness.

9. _____ is the process of creating immunity by introducing a mild antigen into the body.

True or False

1. Histamine can increase the inflammatory response.

2. The digestive system is normally filled with bacteria that would cause disease if the integrity of the bowel were compromised.

3. Gram-positive bacteria cause disease while gram-negative bacteria are harmless.

4. Chronic or recurring arthritis, almost always affecting the knees, may be a consequence of Lyme disease that occurs years after the infecting bite.

5. Tuberculosis is currently a significant health threat in the United States.

6. The more often that bacteria encounter an antibiotic, the more likely it is that they will become resistant to that antibiotic.

7. Viruses are the largest of all disease-causing pathogens.

8. A "yeast infection" is the result of a naturally occurring fungal organism that has multiplied to excessive amounts.

9. Flukes most commonly occur as a result of exposure in a hospital.

10. Aggressive treatment of the common cold includes the administration of antibiotics.

Multiple Choice

1. Which of the following barriers against pathogens does NOT include a chemical component?
   a. skin
   b. saliva
   c. tears
   d. vaginal secretions

2. Which of the following is NOT one of the links in the chain of infection?
   a. pathogen
   b. reservoir
   c. means of transmission
   d. antibody

3. Which of the following is NOT one of the common "portals of entry"?
   a. skin penetration
   b. inhalation
   c. ingestion
   d. injection

4. The immunological defender known as the "big eater" is:
   a. neutrophils
   b. lymphocytes
   c. macrophages
   d. T cells

5. The type of lymphocyte that produces antibodies is:
   a. a helper T cell
   b. a killer T cell
   c. a suppresser T cell
   d. a B cell

6. The second phase of the inflammatory response is:
   a. recognition of the invading pathogen
   b. amplification of defenses
   c. attack
   d. slowdown

7. A reaction by the body's immune system to a harmless substance like dust is:
   a. immunity
   b. an antigen
   c. an allergy
   d. all of the above

8. The smallest pathogens are:
   a. bacteria
   b. fungi
   c. viruses
   d. protozoa

9. Mononucleosis is caused by the virus:
   a. herpes
   b. varicella-zoster
   c. cytomegalovirus
   d. Epstein-Barr

10. A good way to strengthen the immune system is to:
    a. use antihistamines regularly
    b. request annual antibiotic treatment
    c. manage stress effectively
    d. change to a low-fiber diet

SAMPLE TEST QUESTIONS ANSWER KEY

Completion

1. skin (p. 462)
2. host (p. 461)
3. reservoir (p. 460)
4. entry (p. 460)
5. lymphocytes (p. 463)
6. histamine (p. 463)
7. recognition of invading pathogen (p. 464)
8. immunity (p. 464)
9. immunization (p. 466)
10. allergy (p. 468)

True or False

1. T (p. 463)
2. T (p. 469)
3. F (p. 470)
4. T (p. 470)
5. T (p. 471)
6. T (p. 472)
7. F (p. 472)
8. T (p. 476)
9. F (p. 477)
10. F (p. 476)

Multiple Choice

1. a (p. 462)
2. d (p. 460)
3. d (p. 460)
4. c (p. 463)
5. d (p. 463)
6. b (p. 464)
7. c (p. 468)
8. c (p. 472)
9. d (p. 474)
10. c (pp. 478–479)

Turn to the back of the Study Guide, and complete Wellness Worksheets 67–70.

Chapter 18
Sexually Transmitted Diseases

LEARNING OBJECTIVES

As a result of reading Chapter 18 in the textbook and completing the activities in this Study Guide, you should be able to do the following:

1. Discuss the concept of responsible attitudes toward prevention, diagnosis, and treatment of sexually transmitted diseases (STDs).

2. Describe the cause, symptoms (for both men and women), diagnosis, treatment, and consequences of the following major sexually transmitted diseases:
   a. HIV infection/AIDS
   b. chlamydia
   c. gonorrhea
   d. pelvic inflammatory disease (PID)
   e. genital warts
   f. genital herpes
   g. hepatitis B
   h. syphilis

3. Explain how the HIV virus is transmitted, identify the high-risk behaviors for HIV infection, and name the steps individuals can take to protect themselves.

4. Identify several strategies that people may use to reduce the likelihood of HIV transmission and other STDs.

5. Explain why testing, for someone who may have contracted the HIV virus, is an important step for both the person being tested and others.

6. Identify the symptoms of chlamydia and gonorrhea in men and women.

7. Define pelvic inflammatory disease (PID); describe its causes and consequences.

8. Describe the long-term effects of genital warts and herpes.

9. Identify the modes of transmission, symptoms, and customary treatment for hepatitis B.

10. Describe the three stages of syphilis and how syphilis is treated.

11. Discuss the effects of less serious STDs: trichomoniasis, pubic lice, and scabies.

12. Define abstinence and explain why it is the most effective preventive approach to STDs.

TERMINOLOGY

You should be able to define the following key terms:

acquired immune deficiency syndrome (AIDS)
acyclovir
antibody
asymptomatic
Bartholin's glands
blood transfusions
casual contact
CD4 T Cell
chancres
chlamydia
Chlamydia trachomatis
condom
congenital syphilis
dormancy
ELISA (enzyme-linked immunosorbent assay) test
epididymitis
genital herpes
genital self-examination (women/men)
genital warts (condyloma)
gonococcal conjunctivitis
gonorrhea
hemophilia
hepatitis
herpes
herpes simplex, type I
herpes simplex, type II
HIV antibody test
HIV infection
HIV-positive
human herpes virus 6 (HHV 6)
human immunodeficiency virus (HIV)
human papillomavirus (HPV)
immune system
incubation period

jaundice
Kaposi's sarcoma
late syphilis
latent syphilis
Neisseria gonorrhea
nucleoside analog
opportunistic infection
oral sex
pelvic inflammatory disease (PID)
penicillin
pentamidine
Pneumocystis carinii pneumonia (PCP)
podophyllin
primary syphilis
protease inhibitor
pubic lice ("crabs")
safer sex
scabies
secondary syphilis
seroconversion
sexually active
sexually transmitted disease (STD)
spermicide
syphilis
Treponema pallidum
Trichomonas vaginalis
trichomoniasis
unprotected sex
urethritis
vaginal sex
varicella-zoster
vertical transmission
virus
Western blot
yeast infection

MAJOR POINTS/ISSUES

1. Taking charge of your health includes having responsible attitudes toward prevention, diagnosis, and treatment of sexually transmitted diseases.

2. The major STDs are serious in themselves, cause serious complications if untreated, and/or pose risks to a fetus or newborn. These diseases include: HIV infection, hepatitis, syphilis, chlamydia, gonorrhea, herpes, and genital warts.

3. The human immunodeficiency virus (HIV), affects the immune system, taking over the cells that control the body's system of defense against infection. HIV-positive people who develop AIDS are susceptible to infections, especially *Pneumocystis carinii* pneumonia, Kaposi's sarcoma, tuberculosis, and meningitis.

4. HIV infection is an incurable sexually transmitted disease. Two main types of antiviral drugs used to treat HIV infection are nucleoside analogs and protease inhibitors. Scientists predict it will take at least 5 more years to develop an effective vaccine.

5. The HIV virus is transmitted through the exchange of body fluids, including blood, semen, and vaginal fluid. This exchange is most likely to occur during sexual activity, by sharing contaminated needles, and through blood transfusions if the blood supply is contaminated. The time between initial infection and onset of symptoms may range from 2 to 20 years, with an average of 11 years for adults.

6. HIV infection is not spread through casual contact.

7. Preventive behaviors to avoid contact with contaminated body fluids reduce the risk of contracting HIV. For people who are sexually active, preventive behaviors include limiting sexual partners, preferably to one uninfected person who also prefers a monogamous relationship; use of latex condoms during sexual activity; and avoiding sexual contact that could cause cuts or tears in the skin or tissue. People who use IV drugs should not share intravenous needles or anything that might have blood on it.

8. Persons who have engaged in high-risk behavior should be tested for the HIV virus. It is important to know if the HIV virus is present so that passing on the virus to others can be avoided, those who may have already come in contact with the virus can be notified and tested, and early treatment, which often lengthens life, can begin.

9. Hepatitis is an inflammation of the liver, usually caused by one of three viruses. Hepatitis A is the mildest form, usually transmitted by food or water. Hepatitis B is found in all body fluids and is easily transmitted through sexual contact or from contact with blood-contaminated articles. Hepatitis C was once the leading cause of hepatitis following blood transfusions, but blood-supply screening has reduced that risk dramatically.

10. Syphilis is a serious sexually transmitted disease that, if left untreated, can cause central nervous system damage, paralysis, mental degeneration, and death. It follows three distinct stages.

11. Chlamydia is the most prevalent bacterial infection in the United States. The disease is especially dangerous for women because the symptoms are often not noticed and, if chlamydia is undetected for two months or more, it can lead to pelvic inflammatory disease and permanent infertility.

12. Gonorrhea, if untreated, can cause pelvic inflammatory disease and infertility in women, epididymitis and sterility in men, dermatitis, and arthritis. Symptoms for men usually include a noticeable yellowish discharge, but gonorrhea is often asymptomatic in women.

13. Pelvic inflammatory disease (PID), usually a result of untreated chlamydia or gonorrhea, is the major cause of infertility in young women.

14. Genital warts, which are caused by the human papillomavirus and are a highly contagious STD, have been associated with cervical cancer.

15. There are six different viruses in the herpes family, with herpes types I and II, HHV 6, and cytomegalovirus considered sexually transmissible. Herpes is considered a serious STD because of its extremely high incidence and because, unless precautions are taken at birth, it can be transmitted to the baby. There is no cure for herpes, but treatments to reduce pain, avoid secondary infection, and prevent further spread of the infection have improved the outlook for those with herpes.

16. Less serious sexually transmitted diseases include trichomoniasis, a protozoal infection, and pubic lice and scabies, parasitic infections.

17. For all STDs, avoiding sexual contact until healing is complete and following the entire course of treatment, even after symptoms have disappeared, is extremely important.

18. Preventing STDs is each individual's responsibility.

19. All STDs are preventable; the key is practicing responsible sexual behaviors, which requires planning. Those who are sexually active are safest with one mutually faithful uninfected partner. Using a latex condom helps protect against STDs. Use of a diaphragm or cervical cap can provide additional protection.

20. To prevent HIV and other STDs, make careful choices about sexual activity, do not share intravenous drug needles, and participate in STD prevention education programs. All of these actions reduce your risk of contracting a sexually transmitted disease.

SAMPLE TEST QUESTIONS

Completion

1. The leading cause of death of American men in the age group 25–44 and the third leading cause of death for women in the same age group is _____.

2. Among developed nations, the country with the highest rate of STDs is _____.

3. The average asymptomatic period for HIV infected adults in the U.S. is _____ years.

4. The most common means of HIV exposure in the United States have been sexual activity and _____.

5. The confirming laboratory test for HIV infection is the _____.

6. AZT belongs to a category of drugs called _____.

7. Use of a _____ condom provides a high level of protection against HIV.

8. The most common cause of epididymitis is _____.

9. A major complication for infected women untreated for gonorrhea or chlamydia is

    _____.

10. The cause of genital warts is _____ (HPV).

True or False

1. Genital warts are usually diagnosed with blood tests.

2. Once a person has genital herpes, symptoms will always be clearly observable.

3. If a baby is infected with herpesvirus by her mother, the infection will usually occur long before the birth.

4. Herpes infections are cured with the drug acyclovir.

5. Once a person is infected with syphilis, a person will be contagious forever, unless treated.

6. Pubic lice is another name for crabs.

7. Almost all sexually transmitted diseases can be asymptomatic for long periods of time.

8. Results of home HIV testing are reported to state authorities.

9. By age 21, 25% of all college students have contracted a sexually transmitted disease.

10. The riskiest sexual behavior, related to HIV transmission, is anal intercourse.

Multiple Choice

1. Which of the following nations has the highest rate of STDs?
    a. Sweden
    b. Denmark
    c. Holland
    d. United States

2. Currently, it is estimated that the longest time between HIV infection and onset of symptoms is about _____ years.
    a. 2
    b. 11
    c. 15
    d. 20

3. Which of the following may produce trauma that can increase risk of HIV transmission?
    a. enema prior to anal intercourse
    b. excessive use of spermicide
    c. rough intercourse
    d. all of the above

4. Which of the following is "vertical transmission" of HIV?
   a. mother-to-child transmission
   b. transmission by injection
   c. heterosexual transmission
   d. homosexual transmission

5. The rate of AIDS is highest among:
   a. teens
   b. African Americans
   c. Hispanics
   d. whites

6. The likelihood that a baby born to an untreated HIV-positive woman will also become HIV-positive is:
   a. 25%
   b. 50%
   c. 75%
   d. 100%

7. Among men under the age 35, the most frequent cause of epididymitis is:
   a. gonorrhea
   b. chlamydia
   c. syphilis
   d. pubic lice

8. Which of the following medications is NOT effective against chlamydia?
   a. tetracycline
   b. doxycycline
   c. penicillin
   d. erythromycin

9. Human papillomavirus causes:
   a. chlamydia
   b. gonorrhea
   c. genital warts
   d. pubic lice

10. Chancres appear during which stage of syphilis?
    a. primary
    b. secondary
    c. latent
    d. late

SAMPLE TEST QUESTIONS ANSWER KEY

Completion

1. acquired immunodeficiency syndrome (p. 486)
2. United States (p. 486)
3. 11 (p. 489)
4. injecting drug use (p. 489)
5. Western blot (p. 492)
6. nucleoside analogs (p. 493)
7. latex (p. 497)
8. chlamydia (p. 498)
9. pelvic inflammatory disease (PID) (p. 500)
10. human papillomavirus (p. 501)

True or False

1. F (p. 501)
2. F (p. 503)
3. F (p. 503)
4. F (p. 503)
5. F (pp. 504–505)
6. T (p. 505)
7. T (p. 507)
8. F (p. 494)
9. T (p. 502)
10. T (p. 497)

Multiple Choice

1. d (p. 486)
2. d (p. 489)
3. d (p. 489)
4. a (p. 491)
5. b (p. 491)
6. a (p. 491)
7. b (p. 498)
8. c (p. 499)
9. c (p. 501)
10. a (p. 505)

Turn to the back of the Study Guide, and complete Wellness Worksheets 71–72.

Chapter 19
Aging: A Vital Process

LEARNING OBJECTIVES

As a result of reading Chapter 19 in the textbook and completing the activities in this Study Guide, you should be able to do the following:

1. List strategies for healthful aging.

2. Explain the physical, social, and mental changes that may accompany aging, and discuss how people can best confront these changes.

3. Compare different theories of the causes of aging.

4. Describe practical considerations of older adults, including housing, finances, health care, and transportation.

5. Discuss the relationship between lifestyle before the elderly years and health during the elderly years.

6. List the benefits of exercise and a healthy diet for the aging process.

7. Discuss the myth of older adults as a dependent population.

8. Make suggestions for more fully utilizing the wisdom and abilities of the older segment of society.

9. Identify the reasonable expectations children may have in terms of responsibilities for caring for their aging parents.

10. Identify the community resources that older adults may depend upon in solving the unique challenges of aging.

11. Be able to describe the special challenges faced by the aging, regarding access to and payment for health care.

TERMINOLOGY

You should be able to define the following key terms:

"age proofing"
Alzheimer's disease
arthritis
biological aging
cataracts
cerebral cortex
dementia

dendrite
fluid intelligence
geriatrician
gerontologist
glaucoma
hormone replacement therapy (HRT)
life expectancy

life span
Medicaid
Medicare
menopause
neuron

osteoporosis
pension
periodontitis
presbyopia
Social Security

1. People who take charge of their health in youth have greater control over the physical and mental aspects of aging.

2. Biological aging includes all the normal, progressive, irreversible changes to one's body that begin at birth and continue until death. Changes of circumstance, relocating, death of a spouse, retirement, and so on, are occurrences that affect aging.

3. Successful aging requires preparation.

4. Many characteristics traditionally considered to be consequences of aging are due rather to neglect and abuse of body and mind.

5. Exercise throughout life enhances physical and mental health and may prevent deterioration of fluid intelligence.

6. A varied, balanced diet with attention to lower caloric intake promotes health at every age; obesity leads to premature aging.

7. Alcohol and tobacco use impair bodily function and may cause irreversible damage. Overdependence on medications can mimic disease.

8. Regular physical examinations can help detect conditions that may shorten life if left untreated.

9. Aging results from biochemical processes that are not fully understood. Some of the common changes associated with aging can often be prevented, delayed, lessened, or even reversed through good health habits.

10. Planning for social changes, including financial planning for retirement, is key for successful aging. Financial planning is more likely to be critical for women, who are covered by pension plans less often than men are.

11. Anticipating and accommodating the physical changes of aging, including arthritis and declines in hearing and vision, can lead to greater enjoyment.

12. Psychological and mental changes that may occur with aging include forgetfulness, dementia, and grief.

13. Life expectancy, defined as the average length of time we can expect to live, has risen dramatically in the 1900s, with women generally living longer than men.

14. No existing theory of aging accommodates all the facts, and it may be that aging is caused by a variety of different processes and affected by a variety of factors, both environmental and biological.

15. Significantly extended life spans would bring great social changes, the implications of which would necessitate changes in governmental policies and changes in attitudes toward the aged on the part of everyone.

16. Many older people are happy, healthy, and self-sufficient. A variety of family and community resources is available to help older adults remain active and independent.

17. Government aid to the elderly includes food stamps, housing subsidies, Social Security, Medicaid, and Medicare. The question of paying for medical care for older adults, as well as for other citizens, is a problem that continues to be of urgent national significance.

18. Older adults represent an underused resource; society needs to learn to consider productivity and capacity to function rather than age, particularly in terms of employment decisions.

SAMPLE TEST QUESTIONS

Completion

1. The normal, progressive, irreversible changes that begin at birth and continue until death are defined as _____ aging.

2. You can prevent, delay, lessen, and even reverse some of the changes associated with aging through good health habits. These collective practices are called "_____ proofing."

3. One's ability to find solutions when faced with new problems seems to be maintained in aging people by the stimulus provided by exercise. This problem-solving ability is called _____ intelligence.

4. Most older tobacco users started smoking before the age of _____.

5. The average number of years a person spends in retirement is _____.

6. Women outlive men by an average of _____ years.

7. Hormone replacement therapy provides protection against some diseases for which the risk would otherwise increase as a woman ages. Two of the most important of these diseases are osteoporosis and _____ disease.

8. It now appears that our maximum potential life span is about _____ to _____ years.

9. The most common form of elder abuse is _____.

10. The segment of the American population for which suicide is most likely is _____.

True or False

1. Many of the characteristics we associate with aging are actually the result of the neglect and abuse of our mind and body.

2. It is essential that exercise become a part of daily living early in life, because starting an exercise program after age 65 is too late to produce much benefit.

3. Alcohol abuse is not a major problem in old age because most people with serious drinking problems die from alcohol abuse or associated events earlier in life.

4. Financial planning for retirement is even more important for women than for men.

5. A person with hearing loss should be spoken to at a normal rate of speech.

6. Hormone replacement therapy protects women against cancer.

7. The primary reason that the average age of death is greater now than in 1900 is because people are living even longer than they did at the beginning of the century.

8. Biological theories of aging explain the breakdown of the body as a result of a decline in the level of free radicals.

9. Most older Americans live in nursing homes.

10. Nursing home care generally costs at least $3500 per month.

Multiple Choice

1. Government aid to the elderly includes all of the following EXCEPT:
   a. food stamps
   b. housing subsidies
   c. Blue Cross/Blue Shield
   d. Medicaid

2. Aging means becoming:
   a. less healthy
   b. less able
   c. less intelligent
   d. different in structure and function over time

3. The health problem LEAST associated with aging is:
   a. deteriorating vision
   b. loss of hearing of high-pitched tones
   c. bone porousness
   d. dental caries

4. Which of the following is NOT a change in eyesight that is likely to occur as you age?
   a. presbyopia
   b. cataracts
   c. near-sightedness
   d. poor night vision

5. Which of the following statements about aging is true?
   a. Requirements for vitamins and minerals are lower for people over age 65.
   b. Glaucoma inevitably leads to blindness.
   c. The ability to hear high-pitched sounds increases with age.
   d. Alcohol and drug abuse are common problems among the elderly.

6. Which of the following is a common form of arthritis?
   a. dendrites
   b. gout
   c. presbyopia
   d. dementia

7. Glaucoma is elevated pressure in the:
   a. aorta
   b. cerebral circulatory system
   c. legs
   d. eye

8. Gerontologists specialize in treatment of
   a. skin conditions
   b. cancer
   c. problems of the elderly
   d. neurological conditions

9. Which of the following is NOT associated with smoking?
   a. premature skin wrinkling
   b. premature balding
   c. hearing loss
   d. heart disease

10. Approximately four million Americans have Alzheimer's disease. That number is expected to increase by _____ times in the next 20 years.
    a. 2
    b. 3
    c. 4
    d. 5

SAMPLE TEST QUESTIONS ANSWER KEY

Completion

1. biological (p. 516)
2. age (p. 517)
3. fluid (p. 517)
4. 25 (p. 520)
5. 17 (p. 520)
6. 7 (p. 521)
7. heart (p. 523)
8. 100, 110 (p. 526)
9. neglect (p. 531)
10. older white men (p. 525)

True or False

1. T (p. 516)
2. F (p. 518)
3. F (p. 520)
4. T (p. 521)
5. T (p. 522)
6. F (p. 523)
7. F (p. 526)
8. F (p. 526)
9. F (p. 527)
10. T (p. 530)

Multiple Choice

1. c (p. 531)
2. d (p. 516)
3. d (pp. 521–523)
4. c (pp. 522–523)
5. d (p. 520)
6. b (p. 523)
7. d (p. 522)
8. c (p. 532)
9. c (p. 520)
10. b (p. 525)

Turn to the back of the Study Guide, and complete Wellness Worksheets 73–74.

Chapter 20
Dying and Death

LEARNING OBJECTIVES

As a result of reading Chapter 20 in the textbook and completing the activities in this Study Guide, you should be able to do the following:

1. Explain the physical, spiritual, social, and emotional dimensions of death.

2. Discuss legal considerations in planning for death, including wills, advance directives, and organ donation.

3. Understand personal considerations in preparing for death, such as deciding where to die, deciding whether to prolong life, and making funeral arrangements.

4. Describe the stages or process that a dying person may go through.

5. List ways you can support a person who is dying.

5. Explain the grieving process and ways you can support a person who has suffered a loss.

TERMINOLOGY

You should be able to define the following key terms:

active euthanasia
advance directive
autopsy
brain death
causality
cellular death
clinical death
coroner
durable power of attorney for health care
dying
electroencephalogram (EEG)
embalming
funeral
grief/mourning
hospice
intestate
irreversibility of death
lethal injection
life-support systems
living will
"medical Miranda warning"

memorial society
natural death
noncorporeal continuity
nonfunctionality
obituary
palliative care
passive euthanasia
Patient Self Determination Act
persistent vegetative state
physician-assisted death
power of attorney
psychological autopsy
suicide
survivor
terminal illness
testator
Uniform Donor Card
universality of death
unnatural death
will

MAJOR POINTS AND ISSUES

1. There are several criteria by which death is determined. Death may be labeled as brain death, clinical death, and cellular death.

2. One of the challenges of coming to terms with death is that no completely satisfactory answer can be provided to everyone.

3. The age of 10 is the point beyond which almost all children understand death to be universal and irreversible.

4. Coming to terms with one's mortality is healthy.

5. Important decisions related to death include making a will.

6. Hospice care facilitates a person's home death so she/he can remain in familiar and comfortable surroundings.

7. Hospice care is palliative (non-curative) care ordinarily provided by interdisciplinary teams of health care professionals who assist family members in caring for a dying loved one at home.

8. Terminal patients can legally give the responsibility for making important decisions to others by using a power of attorney.

9. Active euthanasia facilitates death through acts of commission. Passive euthanasia facilitates death through acts of omission.

10. Burial and cremation are the customary practices in American culture for disposing of a body after death.

11. Funerals and related events assist survivors in resolving their grief.

12. There are many common responses to one's imminent death, including denial, anger, and depression. Some dying people embrace the prospect of their death and what they anticipate will happen to them after the end of their physical life.

13. Supporting a dying or bereaved person includes being willing to listen and recognizing that people react differently when faced with this challenge.

14. Deceiving children about the circumstances of death or excluding them from death-related rituals is not helpful. Supporting bereaved children should include involving them in the family's grieving experience.

SAMPLE TEST QUESTIONS

Completion

1. Lack of receptivity and response to external stimuli, absence of spontaneous muscular movement and breathing, absence of observable reflexes, and absence of brain activity are the criteria for _____.

2. The gradual process that takes place when the heartbeat, respiration, and brain activity have stopped is called _____.

3. Identifying the thoughts, feelings, and actions of a suicide victim prior to her or his death may be achieved by a _____.

4. A person who dies without a will is said to have died _____.

5. The greatest acceptance of active euthanasia is in this country: _____.

6. Living wills, natural death directives, and durable powers of attorney are known collectively as _____.

7. Medical care that provides comfort, especially pain control, without seeking a cure is called _____ care.

8. The legal authority to act on another person's behalf is called _____.

9. A clinical term for profound unconsciousness accompanied by lack of any normal reflexes, lack of response to external stimuli, and no hope for improvement is _____.

10. Withdrawing or not initiating treatments that could potentially sustain life is sometimes termed _____.

True or False

1. Brain death cannot occur before cellular death.

2. Universality of death and irreversibility of death are the same thing.

3. Dying intestate is the same as dying with a will.

4. Palliative care is for the purpose of curing the patient.

5. The belief that care of dying patients in hospitals was inadequate resulted in hospice care.

6. A power of attorney allows you to legally make decisions for another person.

7. Active euthanasia occurs more often than passive euthanasia.

8. Memorial societies provide funeral services for a profit.

9. The intensity of grief a survivor feels is influenced by the cause of a person's death.

10. An important guide to involving children in funerals or other rituals after a death is in the child's own interest, usually expressed in questions.

Multiple Choice

1. Which of the following is NOT a characteristic of brain death?
   a. unresponsivity
   b. incoherence
   c. flat EEG
   d. no movement

2. Society's unrealistic picture of death can MOST likely be seen in:
   a. television and video games
   b. textbooks
   c. news reporting
   d. popular fiction

3. The testator of a will is the:
   a. attorney who represents the survivors
   b. person making the will
   c. closest living relative
   d. beneficiary of the will

4. A hospice is:
   a. a facility where the dying are isolated from the rest of society
   b. a facility or program that seeks to maximize quality of life for terminally ill patients
   c. a hospital where people are kept alive with expensive equipment
   d. a clinic where terminally ill patients go to test experimental treatments

5. The part of the world in which euthanasia is most accepted by the culture is:
   a. America
   b. China
   c. Australia
   d. the Netherlands

6. Brain death is characterized by:
   a. social isolation
   b. no reflexes
   c. breakdown of metabolic processes
   d. terminal diagnosis

7. The average age at which children begin to develop an adult concept of death is:
   a. 3
   b. 5
   c. 10
   d. 15

8. When someone dies without a will, the state:
   a. distributes the property to the next-of-kin
   b. appoints an administrator from the courts
   c. puts the assets into the public coffers
   d. pays the deceased's creditors before doing anything else

9. Prior to this century, most people died:
   a. in a hospice
   b. at home
   c. in a hospital or nursing home
   d. under the direct care of a physician

10. The patients receiving the MOST attention from hospices have been:
    a. patients with AIDS
    b. terminally ill children
    c. patients receiving technologically advanced treatments
    d. terminally ill cancer patients

SAMPLE TEST QUESTIONS ANSWER KEY

Completion

1. brain death (p. 538)
2. cellular death (p. 538)
3. psychological autopsy (p. 540)
4. intestate (p. 543)
5. the Netherlands (p. 546)
6. advance directives (p. 546)
7. palliative (p. 544)
8. power of attorney (p. 544)
9. persistent vegetative state (p. 544)
10. passive euthanasia (p. 546)

True or False

1. F (p. 538)
2. F (p. 540)
3. F (p. 543)
4. F (p. 544)
5. T (p. 544)
6. T (p. 544)
7. F (p. 546)
8. F (p. 551)
9. T (p. 554)
10. T (p. 557)

Multiple Choice

1. b (p. 538)
2. a (p. 540)
3. b (p. 543)
4. b (p. 544)
5. d (p. 546)
6. b (p. 538)
7. c (p. 539)
8. b (p. 543)
9. b (p. 543)
10. d (p. 544)

Turn to the back of the Study Guide, and complete Wellness Worksheets 75–77.

Chapter 21
Medical Self-Care:
Skills for the Health Care Consumer

LEARNING OBJECTIVES

As a result of reading Chapter 21 in the textbook and completing the activities in this Study Guide, you should be able to do the following:

1. Describe your role as your own primary health care provider.

2. Explain the self-care decision-making process, including how to decide whether to see a physician.

3. Discuss options for self-treatment.

4. Explain the patient-physician partnership, including how to communicate effectively with a health care professional.

5. Describe how medical problems are diagnosed, tested, and treated, and list ways that patients can participate fully in each step.

6. Describe medical tests presently available and explain the benefits of home tests.

7. Name the conditions that require immediate medical treatment.

8. Name several nondrug options for self-care and make a case for choosing a nondrug option over a medication.

9. Describe precautions that need to be taken whenever over-the-counter medications are used.

10. Name the common problems associated with the use of prescription drugs and make suggestions for eliminating those problems.

11. Explain the importance of a second opinion and describe how to get one.

TERMINOLOGY

You should be able to define the following key terms:

antibiotic
consumer
diagnostic process
drug interactions
elective surgery

endoscopy
false negative
false positive
generic drug
home medical tests

medical history
morbidity rate
mortality rate
nondrug options
outpatient
over-the-counter (OTC) medication
persistent
physical examination
physician-patient partnership
prescription medications
provider
recurrent
review of systems
second opinion

self-assessment
self-care
self-diagnosis
self-medication
self-treatment
severe
side effects
social history
symptoms
trauma
treatment options
unusual
vital signs

MAJOR POINTS AND ISSUES

1. There are several skills necessary for effective medical self-care. They include observation of your own symptoms, knowing when to seek professional advice, the ability to self-treat when appropriate, and being able to develop a partnership with your physician.

2. Most home medicine chests are overstocked. Only a few supplies are essential, and a limited supply of additional items depend on your family's personal needs.

3. There are several steps to facilitating effective communication with your physician. They include preparing for the visit ahead of time by noting descriptions of the nature and duration of your symptoms, preparing written questions about your condition, identifying your current medications, and providing relevant medical records, if not otherwise available.

4. The primary steps in the diagnostic process are taking the medical history, conducting the physical examination, and medical testing.

5. The decision to have surgery is an important one and should be made with a full understanding of the risks and side effects of the surgery and nonsurgical alternatives.

6. Prescription medications are an important medical tool and should be used with care. The patient should know when to take the medication, whether to take it with food or before or after eating, and if alcohol should be avoided.

SAMPLE TEST QUESTIONS

Completion

1. Medications that are available without a prescription are known as _____ drugs.

2. _____ drugs are less expensive alternatives to brand name drugs.

3. Research reveals that physicians allow patients to talk for only about
    _____ before interrupting them.

4. If the only tool physicians had to diagnose patients was the patients' descriptions of
    their symptoms, they could still provide a correct diagnosis in more than
    _____ percent of all cases.

5. The most powerful tool in the physician-patient partnership is the
    _____.

6. The most important part of the diagnostic process is usually the _____.

7. The three steps of the diagnostic process are (1) _____,
    (2) _____, and (3) _____.

8. The percentage of medical tests that are probably unnecessary: _____%.

9. Surgeries that a patient can schedule are called _____.

10. Risk of death is defined as the _____ rate.

True or False

1. Originally, the only tool available for home medical testing was the thermometer.

2. "Watchful waiting" will usually result in symptoms becoming more difficult to treat
    when you finally present yourself to a physician.

3. Nondrug options should usually be avoided.

4. Generic medications are usually less expensive than brand name medications.

5. The changing nature of medicine has resulted in physicians spending more time
    listening to patients.

6. Most conditions can be accurately diagnosed by a patient's description of the
    symptoms.

7. The first and most important element of the diagnostic process is the physical
    examination.

8. The majority of medical tests are unnecessary.

9. One in 20 patients admitted to hospitals are there for treatment of a reaction to a drug.

10. Drug patents usually last for five years.

Multiple Choice

1. Which of the following is a necessary skill for effectively managing one's own health?
   a. being a good observer of your own body
   b. possessing detailed knowledge of prescription drugs
   c. knowing the costs of medical tests
   d. being on the defensive with your physician

2. Which of the following is the most common mistake patients make?
   a. Patients ask too many questions.
   b. Patients throw away medications before they expire.
   c. Patients don't seek professional help at the appropriate time.
   d. Patients telephone physicians for medical advice.

3. All of the following are characteristics of symptoms that suggest the need to see a physician immediately EXCEPT:
   a. severe
   b. persistent
   c. recurring
   d. responsive to over-the-counter medications

4. Which of the following is a medical emergency?
   a. persistent cough
   b. shortness of breath
   c. diarrhea
   d. indigestion

5. Headache pain may be relieved by:
   a. ice packs
   b. neck exercises
   c. massage
   d. all of the above

6. You are most likely to save money by:
   a. using over-the-counter medications
   b. using brand name drugs
   c. using generic drugs
   d. not using medications, even when prescribed

7. Preparation for visiting your doctor should include all of the following EXCEPT:
   a. writing questions for the doctor
   b. increasing your insurance coverage
   c. making a list of current medications
   d. providing medical records not otherwise available to your doctor

8. How much time, on average, does the doctor give the patient to talk, before interrupting?
   a. as long as needed
   b. less than 30 seconds
   c. less than a minute
   d. more than two minutes

9. At the end of a medical visit with your doctor it is NOT necessary to:
   a. repeat key points
   b. know the follow-up plan
   c. give your physician feedback
   d. ask the doctor to make another appointment for you

10. Which of the following is true of medical tests in America?
    a. The annual cost of medical testing averages $300 per year per person.
    b. The average number of tests is more than 40 for each American.
    c. Most medical tests are unnecessary.
    d. All of the above are true.

SAMPLE TEST QUESTIONS ANSWER KEY

Completion

1. over-the-counter (p. 567)
2. generic (p. 568)
3. 18 seconds (p. 572)
4. 70 (p. 572)
5. question (p. 572)
6. medical history (p. 572)
7. medical history, physical examination, medical testing (p. 574)
8. 25 (p. 575)
9. elective (p. 578)
10. mortality (p. 578)

True or False

1. T (p. 564)
2. F (p. 566)
3. F (p. 566)
4. T (p. 568)
5. F (p. 572)
6. T (p. 572)
7. F (p. 574)
8. F (p. 575)
9. T (p. 577)
10. F (p. 578)

Multiple Choice

1. a (p. 564)
2. c (p. 565)
3. d (p. 566)
4. b (p. 566)
5. d (p. 566)
6. c (p. 568)
7. b (pp. 571–572)
8. b (p. 572)
9. d (p. 574)
10. b (p. 575)

Turn to the back of the Study Guide, and complete Wellness Worksheets 78–81.

Chapter 22
The Health Care System

LEARNING OBJECTIVES

As a result of reading Chapter 22 in the textbook and completing the activities in this Study Guide, you should be able to do the following:

1. Define the term conventional health care.

2. Describe the services provided by five common independent practitioners.

3. Explain the advantages and disadvantages of using different types of health care facilities.

4. Give examples of allied health care providers.

5. Describe how to evaluate and choose a primary care physician.

6. Differentiate between conventional and unconventional practitioners and provide examples of each.

7. For each of the following unconventional practices, describe the philosophy underlying the practice, the therapies that are usually conducted, the medical benefits claimed, and the risks associated with treatment.
   a. Chiropractic
   b. Acupuncture
   c. Homeopathy
   d. Naturopathy
   e. Ayurvedic medicine
   f. Clinical ecology

8. Describe ways to protect oneself from health quackery.

9. Describe the current system of health care payments in the United States.

10. Describe two basic types of health insurance, including the usual services provided by each type.

11. Identify the government programs established for the provision of medical services and the population groups served by each.

12. Discuss the advantages and disadvantages of each of the following types of health insurance: point of service plans, health maintenance organizations, and preferred provider organizations.

13. Describe the differences between traditional and managed care.

14. List the factors that need to be considered when choosing a health insurance policy.

15. List questions to ask in evaluating different health insurance plans.

TERMINOLOGY

You should be able to define the following key terms:

acupressure (shiatsu)
acupuncture
allied health care provider
alternative medicine
Ayurvedic medicine
basic coverage
capitation
chiropractic
clinical ecology
coinsurance provision
comprehensive major medical insurance
conventional health care
conventional practitioners
deductible clause
dentist
"dread disease" policies
group policies
health insurance
health maintenance organization (HMO)
homeopathy

hypersensitivity
independent practitioner
individual policies
major medical insurance
managed-care plan
Medicaid
medical doctor
medical specialties
Medicare
meridians
naturopathy
optometrist
osteopathic physician
outpatient
podiatrist
point-of-service (POS) plan
preferred provider organization (PPO)
prepaid group plans
quackery
unconventional practitioners

MAJOR POINTS/ISSUES

1. Conventional health care is the prevention, diagnosis, and treatment of disease based on currently accepted scientific information.

2. Medical doctors have degrees from accredited medical schools and are licensed to administer medical and surgical treatment; specialists have additional training and can become board-certified. Other independent practitioners include osteopathic physicians, podiatrists, optometrists, and dentists.

3. Other conventional health practitioners who are licensed to provide specific types of care are allied health care providers, including registered nurses, licensed vocational nurses, nurse-practitioners, certified nurse-midwives, dietitians, dental hygienists, physical therapists, occupational therapists, laboratory technicians, and X ray technicians.

4. Things to look for in a primary care physician include staff affiliation with a hospital connected with a medical school or residency program, current credentials, and recommendations. A "get-acquainted" visit is helpful for making a final evaluation.

5. Unconventional practice consists of philosophies or methods that clash with accepted knowledge or are unproven and unlikely. Unorthodox practitioners sometimes help people by giving them attention, helping them to relieve stress, and/or persuading them to adopt healthier living habits; but reliance on unscientific practitioners may delay effective care and often involves financial exploitation.

6. Common unconventional approaches to health care in the United States are chiropractic, homeopathy, naturopathy, acupuncture, Ayurvedic medicine, and clinical ecology.

7. Protection against medical quackery is ensured by maintaining a level of suspicion and by reading or seeking out information from qualified groups.

8. Health care in the United States is currently financed by a combination of patient out-of-pocket payments, private and public insurance payments, and public assistance.

9. Health insurance enables people to budget in advance for health care costs that could otherwise be ruinous. Since medical care has become a major expense, health insurance is important for almost everyone.

10. There are two basic types of health insurance coverage: basic health insurance covers expenses for hospital, surgical, and medical care; major medical insurance protects against medical expenses resulting from prolonged illness or injury.

11. Group policies, most often offered through employers, usually provide more coverage and cost less than individual policies.

12. Government programs to provide medical care for those who cannot afford insurance include Medicaid, a state-run federally subsidized program, and Medicare, a program for those 65 and over and the chronically disabled.

13. Prepaid group plans have been developed to help reduce the cost of medical care. These plans include health maintenance organizations, programs wherein physicians agree to accept a monthly fee per patient or to adhere to a lowered fee schedule. Patients are limited to member physicians. Preferred provider organizations are programs in which participating physicians and hospitals agree to accept fixed fees that are usually 15 to 20 percent less than their usual fees.

14. Point-of-service (POS) plans are managed-care plans that cover treatment by an HMO physician but permit the patient to seek treatment elsewhere with a higher copayment.

15. Choosing health insurance can be complicated because plans and contracts vary widely. Overall, group policies are usually best. Choice should depend on services covered, exclusions, deductibles, maximum limits, and choice of care providers.

SAMPLE TEST QUESTIONS

Completion

1. _____ are independent practitioners whose care is limited to problems of feet and legs.

2. Independent practitioners who detect vision problems and eye diseases but do not do surgery are _____.

3. Registered nurses, registered dietitians, psychologists, and social workers are examples of health care professionals who are categorized as _____ providers.

4. The most frequent complaints presented to _____ are back aches and musculoskeletal disorders.

5. A noninvasive application of pressure, similar to acupuncture, is _____.

6. _____ remedies depend on an application principle that is the reverse of the standard dose-response relationship.

7. Two types of insurance policies are basic and _____ medical.

8. Individuals who are chronically disabled or have reached the age of 65 are eligible for _____.

9. HMO is an acronym that stands for _____.

10. Managed-care plans try to discourage overtreatment through the use of _____.

True or False

1. Medical practice and osteopathic practice are essentially the same.

2. The best time to start looking for a physician is when you first become sick.

3. There is strong scientific support for regular chiropractic visits to maintain good health.

4. Meridians are the identifying markers that allow the practitioners of naturopathy to diagnose disease.

5. Homeopathic remedies have remained on the market because of conclusive research that has demonstrated their effectiveness.

6. The government pays for the majority of all health care costs.

7. The advantages of group health insurance policies include broader coverage and lower cost.

8. Medicaid is a health insurance program for people over the age of 65.

9. Point-of-service plans are a type of managed care that allows use of personally selected physicians if the patient accepts responsibility for a larger percentage of the cost of treatment.

10. The Office of Alternative Medicine was created to promote insurance coverage of unconventional health practices.

Multiple Choice

1. Osteopaths are most like:
   a. medical doctors
   b. podiatrists
   c. optometrists
   d. chiropractors

2. Treatment of the feet and legs is the practice of:
   a. naturopathy
   b. homeopathy
   c. podiatry
   d. chiropractic

3. Which of the following is NOT considered an allied health professional?
   a. registered nurse
   b. registered dietitian
   c. podiatrist
   d. social worker

4. Which of the following is LEAST suited to be a primary care physician?
   a. pediatrician
   b. family practice specialist
   c. internal medicine specialist
   d. cardiologist

5. Which of the following is NOT allowed to prescribe drugs distributed by a pharmacist?
   a. dentist
   b. chiropractor
   c. osteopath
   d. medical doctor

6. Shiatsu is another name for:
   a. acupuncture
   b. acupressure
   c. homeopathy
   d. Ayurvedic medicine

7. Which of the following is practiced by a few hundred osteopaths and medical doctors?
   a. clinical ecology
   b. naturopathy
   c. iridology
   d. reflexology

8. Government-provided health insurance for people over the age of 65 is called:
   a. Senior Care
   b. Medicare
   c. Medicaid
   d. Opticare

9. The patient has the greatest personal choice of providers under:
   a. Medicare
   b. point-of-service plans
   c. health maintenance organizations
   d. traditional insurance plans

10. Preferred-provider plans control costs by:
    a. negotiating physician fees that are 15% to 20% lower than customary charges
    b. limiting the types of cases that will be accepted
    c. limiting care to people who are not yet retired
    d. all of the above

SAMPLE TEST QUESTIONS ANSWER KEY

Completion

1. Podiatrists (p. 584)
2. optometrists (p. 584)
3. allied health care (p. 585)
4. chiropractors (p. 587)
5. acupressure (p. 588)
6. Homeopathic (p. 588)
7. major (p. 593)
8. Medicare (p. 593)
9. health maintenance organization (p. 593)
10. "gatekeepers" (p. 594)

True or False

1. T (p. 584)
2. F (p. 586)
3. F (p. 587)
4. F (pp. 588–589)
5. F (p. 588)
6. F (p. 591)
7. T (p. 593)
8. F (p. 593)
9. T (p. 594)
10. F (p. 588)

Multiple Choice

1. a (p. 584)
2. c (p. 584)
3. c (p. 584)
4. d (pp. 585–586)
5. b (p. 589)
6. b (p. 588)
7. a (p. 589)
8. b (p. 593)
9. d (p. 593)
10. a (pp. 593–594)

Turn to the back of the Study Guide, and complete Wellness Worksheets 82–83.

Chapter 23
Personal Safety: Protecting Yourself from Unintentional Injuries and Violence

LEARNING OBJECTIVES

As a result of reading Chapter 23 in the textbook and completing the activities in this Study Guide, you should be able to do the following:

1. Discuss factors that contribute to unintentional injuries.

2. List the most common types of unintentional injuries.

3. Describe strategies for preventing unintentional injuries.

4. Describe factors that contribute to violence and unintentional injuries.

5. Discuss different forms of violence.

6. Discuss how to protect oneself from intentional injuries.

7. List strategies for assisting others in an emergency situation.

TERMINOLOGY

You should be able to define the following key terms:

acquaintance or date rape
air bag
all-terrain vehicle (ATV)
assault
battering
cardiopulmonary resuscitation (CPR)
carpal tunnel syndrome
cumulative trauma disorders (CTDs)
emergency medical services (EMS) system
environmental factors
first aid
gang-related violence
hate crimes
heat cramps
heat exhaustion

Heimlich maneuver
home injuries
homicide
human factors
incest
intentional injury
in-line skates
leisure injuries
motor vehicle injuries
multiple causation theory
Occupational Safety and Health
    Administration (OSHA)
pedestrian safety
personal flotation device (PDF)
physical impairments

psychological factors
rape
repetitive-strain injuries
risk-taking behavior
Rohypnol
safety belts

sexual assault
sexual harassment
statutory rape
unintentional injury
work injuries
years of potential life lost

MAJOR POINTS/ISSUES

1. Engineering, enforcement, and education are the three primary ways to prevent and reduce injuries. Ultimately, it is up to each individual to protect one's self against injuries.

2. Unintentional injuries are a leading cause of death in the United States. Motor vehicle crashes are the leading cause of death of Americans age 1 through 25.

3. Most injuries are caused by a combination of human and environmental factors.

4. Primary contributors to motor vehicle injuries are bad driving, failure to use safety belts, driving while intoxicated, and driving in dangerous environmental conditions.

5. A variety of specific steps can reduce the risk of motor vehicle injuries, including obeying the speed limit, wearing a safety belt, never driving while intoxicated, driving on controlled access highways when possible, and obeying traffic signals.

6. Head injuries are a leading cause of death among riders of bicycles, mopeds, and motorcycles.

7. Home injuries usually involve falls, fires, poisoning, suffocation, and unintentional firearm injuries.

8. Frequent leisure injuries are sports injuries, drowning, boating injuries, injuries that occur on playgrounds, and injuries that occur to users of all-terrain vehicles and in-line skates.

9. There has been a dramatic reduction in the percentage of work-related injuries as a result of implementing recommendations in the workplace similar to those discussed in this chapter.

10. Violence and its consequences have become a major public health concern. Violence includes homicide, sexual assault, domestic violence, suicide, and other types of abuse.

11. A variety of factors contribute to violence including social circumstances, interpersonal factors, alcohol and drug use patterns, and access to firearms.

12. There has been an increase in the number of hate crimes in the United States.

13. Family violence is a serious public health problem and is probably more serious than is indicated by the data because family violence frequently goes unreported.

14. More than 3.5 million rapes occur annually. Women may reduce their risk of being raped by screaming when an assault commences, fighting back, kicking, or claiming to have a sexually transmitted disease.

15. Steps in giving emergency care include making sure the scene is safe for you and the injured person, finding out what happened, conducting a quick examination of the victim, giving emergency first aid, and seeking help.

SAMPLE TEST QUESTIONS

Completion

1. The phrase that describes the difference between one's average life expectancy and age at the time of a premature death is _____.

2. Falls, motor vehicle crashes, and poisonings are all causes of _____ injuries.

3. The three "E's" of injury prevention are _____, _____, and _____.

4. The leading cause of death for Americans between the ages of 1 and 25 is _____.

5. Most _____ only protect auto passengers in head-on collisions.

6. A safety practice important to riders of bicycles, mopeds, and motorcycles is the wearing of _____ .

7. Increased use of computer terminals has resulted in an increase in the number of cases of _____ syndrome.

8. One reason for the high rate of homicide in the United States is the widespread availability of _____.

9. Coerced sexual activity in which the victim knows the rapist is often called _____ rape.

10. A person who sexually pressures someone in a vulnerable or subordinate position is engaging in _____.

True or False

1. Unintentional injuries are the leading cause of death for people under age 45.

2. The primary cause of motor vehicle crashes is bad driving, especially speeding.

3. Airbags cause more injuries than they prevent.

4. Head injuries are the cause of most bicycle-related deaths.

5. Alcohol is a contributing factor in a significant number of pedestrian deaths.

6. More deaths due to falls occur among young people than older people.

7. Most fatal burns occur in the home.

8. The highest drowning rate is among early teens.

9. People under the age of 25 account for almost 50% of the arrests for violent crimes in the United States.

10. Because each situation is different, experts disagree about whether a woman should resist a rapist.

Multiple Choice

1. The LEAST frequent contributor to motor vehicle crashes is:
   a. environmental conditions
   b. alcohol and drug use
   c. poor vehicle condition
   d. bad driving

2. The single factor that could reduce injuries in motor vehicle crashes most is:
   a. having operating airbags in the car
   b. wearing safety belts
   c. not exceeding 40 miles per hour
   d. doing most driving in close proximity to home

3. Which of the following is NOT considered a home injury?
   a. fall
   b. fire
   c. poisoning
   d. bicycle injury

4. Poisoning deaths occur most frequently among which age group?
   a. under 5
   b. 5–9
   c. 10–14
   d. 15 and above

5. The Heimlich maneuver is an appropriate intervention technique in the case of:
   a. poisoning
   b. burns
   c. choking
   d. injuries due to falls

6. Which of the following is NOT considered a leisure injury?
   a. bicycle injury
   b. drowning
   c. in-line skating injury
   d. sports injury

7. What agency seems to have contributed most to a reduction of work-related injuries?
   a. Occupational Safety and Health Administration
   b. Association for Worksite Wellness
   c. National Wellness Association
   d. Food and Drug Administration

8. Carpal tunnel syndrome is a problem of the:
   a. eyes
   b. hands
   c. back
   d. nerves

9. Rates of violence are highest in which region of the United States?
   a. west
   b. east
   c. north central
   d. south

10. Most victims of family violence are:
    a. children
    b. women
    c. men
    d. minorities

SAMPLE TEST QUESTIONS ANSWER KEY

Completion

1. years of potential life lost (p. 602)
2. unintentional (p. 602)
3. engineering, enforcement, education (p. 602)
4. motor vehicle crashes (p. 603)
5. airbags (p. 604)
6. helmets (p. 607)
7. carpal tunnel (p. 614)
8. handguns (p. 615)
9. date or acquaintance (p. 620)
10. sexual harassment (p. 623)

True or False

1. T (p. 602)
2. T (p. 603)
3. F (p. 604)
4. T (p. 607)
5. T (p. 607)
6. F (pp. 607–608)
7. T (p. 609)
8. F (p. 611)
9. T (p. 616)
10. T (p. 621)

Multiple Choice

1. c (p. 603)
2. b (p. 604)
3. d (p. 607)
4. a (p. 609)
5. c (p. 611)
6. a (p. 611)
7. a (p. 613)
8. b (p. 614)
9. a (p. 615)
10. b (p. 618)

Turn to the back of the Study Guide, and complete Wellness Worksheets 84–87.

Chapter 24
Environmental Health

LEARNING OBJECTIVES

As a result of reading Chapter 24 in the textbook and completing the activities in this Study Guide, you should be able to do the following:

1. Describe the methods that are used to deal with the classic environmental concerns of clean water and waste disposal.

2. Discuss the effects of rapid increases in human population, and list factors that may limit or slow world population growth.

3. Describe the short- and long-term effects of air, chemical, and noise pollution and exposure to radiation.

4. Outline strategies that individuals, communities, and nations can take to preserve and restore the environment.

TERMINOLOGY

You should be able to define the following key terms:

acid precipitation	garbage
aerosol sprays	global warming
air pollution	greenhouse effect
asbestos	hazardous waste
asbestosis	heavy metal
biodiversity	herbicides
biological pollutants	insecticides
biomagnification	lead poisoning
bubonic plague	London-type smog
carbon monoxide	Los Angeles-type smog
chemical pollution	Lyme disease
chlorofluorocarbons (CFCs)	noise pollution
cholera	nuclear power
ecosystem	ozone layer
emission control standards	pesticides
emissions	phon
encephalitis	photochemical smog
environmental health	pollutant
fertility rate	pollution
fluoridation	polychlorinated biphenyl (PCB)
food chain	radiation
food inspection	radiation sickness
fossil fuels	radioactive waste

radon
recycle
recycling centers
Rocky Mountain spotted fever
sanitary landfill
septic system
sewage

solid waste
temperature inversion
tinnitus
toxic waste
waste disposal
water pollution

MAJOR POINTS AND ISSUES

1. The historical focus of environmental health has been preventing the spread of infectious diseases via water, waste, food, and rodents and insects. For a variety of reasons the focus of environmental health has become broader.

2. Water is one of the most important requirements for human health, and yet there are few places in the world where there is enough safe drinking water.

3. Population growth is a primary reason for increasing water shortages.

4. Waste generated by humans, from aluminum cans to newspapers, is a significant environmental health issue.

5. The biggest single component of household trash is paper, followed by yard waste.

6. The custom of burying solid waste in landfills has several disadvantages, including cost, space requirements, and the threat of soil contamination.

7. Recycling centers have dramatically reduced the amount of solid waste that ends up in landfills.

8. Although the food distribution system in the United States is very safe, it is estimated that Americans average more than two minor cases of foodborne illness each year.

9. Many illnesses are transmitted to humans from animals. These include encephalitis, Lyme disease, and Rocky Mountain spotted fever.

10. The roots of most threats to the environment can be found in the tremendous growth in world population, which has more than doubled in just the past half century.

11. Factors that may eventually limit the growth in overall population include limited food supplies, limited land and water, and limited energy sources.

12. Air pollution is sufficiently serious to be a threat to human health in the short and long term. Consequences of air pollution include respiratory difficulties and increases in skin cancer due to deterioration of the ozone layer.

13. World energy use patterns contribute significantly to air pollution. Two strategies for controlling energy use are conservation and developing nonpolluting, renewable energy sources.

14. Indoor air pollution includes tobacco smoke, carbon monoxide, formaldehyde gas, and biological pollutants.

15. Common chemical pollutants include asbestos, pesticides, and lead.

16. Radiation from the sun, uranium, nuclear weapons, medical equipment, and even some sources in the home, can be a threat to health, with extreme effects including radiation sickness, chromosome damage, and cancers.

17. A relatively new environmental concern is radon gas, a naturally occurring radioactive gas found in certain soils, rocks, and building materials.

18. Noise pollution is becoming increasingly severe. Continuous exposure to sound levels above 80–85 phons (approximately the level of sound to which you are exposed if surrounded by heavy traffic) can cause permanent hearing loss.

SAMPLE TEST QUESTIONS

Completion

1. The ingredient with which many cities treat their drinking water to reduce dental caries is _____.

2. Typhoid, cholera, and hepatitis A are likely to be contracted as a result of contact with _____ matter.

3. The biggest single component of solid waste generated from homes is _____.

4. In spite of a safe and efficient food distribution system, Americans average _____ episodes of foodborne illness annually.

5. Rocky Mountain spotted fever is an example of an illness transmitted by a/an _____ vector.

6. The world's population has doubled in approximately the past _____ years.

7. The three simultaneous events that are prerequisites to an air pollution emergency are (1) a source of pollution, (2) topographical contributors to the emergency, and (3) a/an _____.

8. Photochemical smog is so characteristic of one city that it is also called _____-type smog.

9. The shield that protects us from the sun's hazardous ultraviolet rays is the
_____ layer.

10. Prolonged exposure to sounds above _____ phons can cause permanent
hearing loss.

True or False

1. Few parts of the world have adequate quantities of safe drinking water.

2. The primary cause of water shortages is evaporation accelerated by ozone depletion.

3. Yard waste is the single largest component of household waste.

4. Recycling centers have failed to reduce the amount of solid waste deposited in
landfills.

5. The safety of the American food distribution system has eradicated foodborne
illness.

6. The world population doubled between 1940 and 1990.

7. London-type smog is the same as photochemical smog.

8. The ozone layer has been destroyed primarily by chlorofluorocarbons.

9. Air pollution can happen indoors and outdoors.

10. Lead poisoning is a serious threat to senior citizens living in older housing.

Multiple Choice

1. The field of environmental health originally grew out of efforts to:
   a. achieve national health objectives
   b. control communicable diseases
   c. counteract the effect of increasing population on the environment
   d. increase the lifespan of residents of underdeveloped countries

2. Municipal water supplies are fluoridated to:
   a. purify the water
   b. reduce dental caries
   c. remove heavy metals from the water
   d. remove lead from the water

3. The biggest single component of household trash (by weight) is:
   a. plastic
   b. aluminum cans
   c. hazardous materials
   d. paper products

4. It is predicted that the world population will stabilize:
   a. at approximately 8 billion people
   b. at approximately 11 billion people
   c. at approximately 15 billion people
   d. only as the result of massive wars and famine

5. Which of the following conditions is NOT a prerequisite for an air pollution emergency?
   a. pollution source
   b. topographical features limiting air currents
   c. temperature inversion
   d. acid precipitation

6. The primary ozone layer depletion occurs over:
   a. North America
   b. Europe
   c. Africa
   d. Antarctica

7. Which of the following is not a fossil fuel?
   a. oil
   b. nuclear power
   c. coal
   d. natural gas

8. Formaldehyde gas is most likely to come from:
   a. environmental tobacco smoke
   b. kerosene heaters
   c. plywood paneling resin
   d. bacteria

9. The body system most seriously threatened by asbestos is:
   a. digestive
   b. cardiovascular
   c. respiratory
   d. nervous

10. Which of the following is the loudest sound one can listen to continuously without damage to hearing?
    a. normal conversation
    b. vacuum cleaner
    c. motorcycle engine
    d. rifle shots

SAMPLE TEST QUESTIONS ANSWER KEY

Completion

1. fluoride (p. 632)
2. fecal (p. 635)
3. paper (p. 635)
4. 2–3 (p. 637)
5. animal (pp. 637–638)
6. 50 (p. 638)
7. temperature inversion (p. 641)
8. Los Angeles (p. 642)
9. ozone (p. 642)
10. 80–85 (p. 649)

True or False

1. T (p. 632)
2. F (p. 634)
3. F (p. 635)
4. F (p. 636)
5. F (p. 637)
6. T (p. 638)
7. F (p. 641)
8. T (p. 643)
9. T (p. 645)
10. F (p. 647)

Multiple Choice

1. b (p. 632)
2. b (p. 632)
3. d (p. 635)
4. b (p. 638)
5. d (p. 641)
6. d (p. 642)
7. b (p. 645)
8. c (p. 645)
9. c (p. 646)
10. b (p. 650)

Turn to the back of the Study Guide, and complete Wellness Worksheets 88–90.

Wellness Worksheets

Name _____ Section _____ Date _____

WELLNESS WORKSHEET 4

Wellness Profile

Fill in your strengths for each of the dimensions of wellness described below. Examples of strengths are listed with each dimension.

Physical wellness: To maintain overall physical health and engage in appropriate physical activity (e.g., stamina, strength, flexibility, healthy body composition).

_____

_____

_____

_____

Emotional wellness: To have a positive self-concept, deal constructively with your feelings, and develop positive qualities (e.g., optimism, trust, self-confidence, determination, persistence, dedication).

_____

_____

_____

_____

Intellectual wellness: To pursue and retain knowledge, think critically about issues, make sound decisions, identify problems, and find solutions (e.g., common sense, creativity, curiosity).

_____

_____

_____

_____

Spiritual wellness: To develop a set of beliefs, principles, or values that give meaning or purpose to one's life; to develop faith in something beyond oneself (e.g., religious faith, service to others).

_____

_____

_____

_____

Interpersonal/social wellness: To develop and maintain meaningful relationships with a network of friends and family members, and to contribute to the community (e.g., friendly, good-natured, compassionate, supportive, good listener).

_____

_____

_____

_____

Environmental wellness: To protect yourself from environmental hazards, and to minimize the negative impact of your behavior on the environment (e.g., carpooling, recycling).

_____

_____

_____

_____

(over)

Insel/Roth, *Core Concepts in Health*, Eighth Edition. © 1998 Mayfield Publishing Company. Chapter 1
Insel et al., *Core Concepts in Health*, Brief Eighth Edition. © 1998 Mayfield Publishing Company. Chapter 1

Next, choose what you believe are your five most important strengths, and record them under "Core Wellness Strengths."

Core Wellness Strengths

1._____

2._____

3._____

4._____

5._____

Finally, mark on the continuums below where you think you fall for each dimension.

Low Level of Wellness	Physical, Psychological, Emotional Symptoms	Change and Growth	High Level of Wellness

Physical wellness

Emotional wellness

Intellectual wellness

Spiritual wellness

Interpersonal/social wellness

Environmental wellness

WELLNESS WORKSHEET 7

Identify Your Stressors

Signals of Stress

To identify sources of stress in your life you must first be able to identify the signals of stress. Put a check next to any of the listed signs that you have experienced in the last month.

Physical Signs

____ Pounding heart
____ Trembling, with nervous tics
____ Grinding of teeth
____ Dry mouth
____ Excessive perspiration
____ Gastrointestinal problems
____ Stiff neck or aching lower back
____ Migraine or tension headaches
____ Frequent colds or low-grade infections
____ Cold hands and feet
____ Allergy or asthma attacks
____ Skin problems (hives, eczema, psoriasis)

Emotional Signs

____ Tendency to be irritable or aggressive
____ Tendency to feel anxious, fearful, or edgy

____ Hyperexcitability, impulsiveness, or emotional instability
____ Depression
____ Frequent feelings of boredom
____ Inability to concentrate
____ Fatigue

Behavioral Signs

____ Increased use of alcohol, tobacco, or other drugs
____ Excessive TV watching
____ Sleep disturbances or excessive sleep
____ Overeating or undereating
____ Sexual problems
____ Crying or yelling
____ Job or school burnout
____ Spouse or child abuse
____ Panic attacks

Possible Stressful Events

Listed below, in order of probable severity of effect, are thirty-five life events you may experience that cause stress. Put a check next to any item that you have experienced recently or expect to experience soon. If you find you have checked several items, take time out to develop and cultivate your coping skills.

____ Death of a close family member
____ Divorce or separation from mate
____ Detention in jail or other institution
____ Major personal injury or illness
____ Death of a close friend
____ Divorce between parents
____ Marriage
____ Being fired from job or expelled from school
____ Retirement
____ Change in health of a family member
____ Pregnancy
____ Being a victim of a crime
____ Sexual difficulties
____ Gaining new family members (through birth, adoption, older person moving in, etc.)
____ New girlfriend or boyfriend
____ Major business or academic readjustment (merger, change of job or major, failing important course)
____ Major change in financial state (a lot worse or a lot better off than before)
____ Taking out a loan or mortgage for school or a major purchase

____ Trouble with parents, spouse, or girlfriend or boyfriend
____ Outstanding personal achievement
____ Graduation
____ First quarter/semester in college
____ Denied admission to program or school
____ Change in living conditions
____ Serious argument with instructor, friend, or roommate
____ Lower grades than expected
____ Major change in working hours or conditions or increased workload at school
____ Major change in recreational, social, or church activities
____ Major change in sleeping or eating habits
____ Denial of admission to required course
____ Taking out a loan for a lesser purchase (e.g., a car, TV, or freezer)
____ Chronic car trouble
____ Change in number of family get-togethers
____ Vacation
____ Minor violation of the law (such as a traffic ticket)

(over)

Insel/Roth, *Core Concepts in Health,* Eighth Edition. © 1998 Mayfield Publishing Company. Chapter 2
Insel et al., *Core Concepts in Health,* Brief Eighth Edition. © 1998 Mayfield Publishing Company. Chapter 2

Weekly Stress Log

Now that you are familiar with the signals of stress, complete the weekly stress log to map patterns in your stress levels and identify sources of stress. Enter a score for each hour of each day according to the ratings listed below.

	A.M.							P.M.												
	6	7	8	9	10	11	12	1	2	3	4	5	6	7	8	9	10	11	12	Average
Monday																				
Tuesday																				
Wednesday																				
Thursday																				
Friday																				
Saturday																				
Sunday																				
Average																				

Ratings

1 = No anxiety; general feeling of well-being
2 = Mild anxiety; no interference with activity
3 = Moderate anxiety; specific signal(s) of stress present
4 = High anxiety; interference with activity
5 = Very high anxiety and panic reactions; general inability to engage in activity

To identify daily or weekly patterns in your stress level, average your stress rating for each hour and each day. For example, if your scores for 6:00 A.M. are 3, 3, 4, 3, and 4, with blanks for Saturday and Sunday, your 6:00 A.M. rating would be 17 ÷ 5, or 3.4. What hours of the day and days of the week are most stressful for you?

Based on these patterns, what are some of the key sources of stress in your life?

Name _____ Section _____ Date _____

WELLNESS WORKSHEET 8

Time Stress Questionnaire

The following list describes time-related difficulties people sometimes experience. Please indicate how often each is a difficulty for you, using the numbers shown:

__0__ **Seldom or never a difficulty for me**

__1__ **Sometimes a difficulty for me**

__2__ **Frequently a difficulty for me**

_____ My time is directed by factors beyond my control

_____ Interruptions

_____ Chronic overload—more to do than time available

_____ Occasional overload

_____ Chronic underload—too little to do in time available

_____ Occasional underload

_____ Alternating periods of overload and underload

_____ Disorganization of my time

_____ Procrastination

_____ Separating home, school, and work

_____ Transition from work or school to home

_____ Finding time for regular exercise

_____ Finding time for daily periods of relaxation

_____ Finding time for friendships

_____ Finding time for family

_____ Finding time for vacations

_____ Easily bored

_____ Saying "yes" when I later wish I had said "no"

_____ Feeling overwhelmed by large tasks over an extended period of time

_____ Avoiding important tasks by frittering away time on less important ones

_____ Feeling compelled to assume responsibilities in groups

_____ Unable to delegate because no one to delegate to

_____ My perfectionism creates delays

_____ I tend to leave tasks unfinished

_____ I have difficulty living with unfinished tasks

_____ Too many projects going at one time

(over)

Insel/Roth, *Core Concepts in Health,* Eighth Edition. © 1998 Mayfield Publishing Company. Chapter 2
Insel et al., *Core Concepts in Health,* Brief Eighth Edition. © 1998 Mayfield Publishing Company. Chapter 2

_____ Getting into time binds by trying to please others too often

_____ I tend to hurry even when it's not necessary

_____ Lose concentration while thinking about other things I have to do

_____ Not enough time alone

_____ Feel compelled to be punctual

_____ Pressure related to deadlines

Scoring

Add your scores and find your rating below.

0–9	Low difficulty with time-related stressors
10–19	Moderate difficulty with time-related stressors
20 or more	High difficulty with time-related stressors

Now go back and underline the five most significant time-related stressors for you. Identify two concrete strategies you can take to help relieve each of these key stressors.

Stressor 1: _____

    1. _____

    2. _____

Stressor 2: _____

    1. _____

    2. _____

Stressor 3: _____

    1. _____

    2. _____

Stressor 4: _____

    1. _____

    2. _____

Stressor 5: _____

    1. _____

    2. _____

SOURCE: Excerpt adapted from Schafer, W. 1996. *Stress Managment for Wellness,* 3d ed. Copyright © 1996 by Holt, Rinehart and Winston. Reprinted by permission of the publisher.

WELLNESS WORKSHEET 9

Life Hassles and Stress

For each of the following experiences, indicate to what degree it has been a part of your life *over the past month* by writing in the appropriate number.

    1 = not at all part of my life
    2 = only slightly part of my life
    3 = distinctly part of my life
    4 = very much part of my life

_____ 1. Disliking your daily activities

_____ 2. Lack of privacy

_____ 3. Disliking your work

_____ 4. Ethnic or racial conflict

_____ 5. Conflicts with in-laws or boyfriend's/girlfriend's family

_____ 6. Being let down or disappointed by friends

_____ 7. Conflict with supervisor(s) at work

_____ 8. Social rejection

_____ 9. Too many things to do at once

_____ 10. Being taken for granted

_____ 11. Financial conflicts with family members

_____ 12. Having your trust betrayed by a friend

_____ 13. Separation from people you care about

_____ 14. Having your contributions overlooked

_____ 15. Struggling to meet your own standards of performance and accomplishment

_____ 16. Being taken advantage of

_____ 17. Not enough leisure time

_____ 18. Financial conflicts with friends or fellow workers

_____ 19. Struggling to meet other people's standards of performance and accomplishment

_____ 20. Having your actions misunderstood by others

_____ 21. Cash-flow difficulties

_____ 22. A lot of responsibilities

_____ 23. Dissatisfaction with work

_____ 24. Decisions about intimate relationship(s)

_____ 25. Not enough time to meet your obligations

_____ 26. Dissatisfaction with your mathematical ability

(over)

Insel/Roth, *Core Concepts in Health,* Eighth Edition. © 1998 Mayfield Publishing Company. Chapter 2
Insel et al., *Core Concepts in Health,* Brief Eighth Edition. © 1998 Mayfield Publishing Company. Chapter 2

_____ 27. Financial burdens

_____ 28. Lower evaluation of your work than you think you deserve

_____ 29. Experiencing high levels of noise

_____ 30. Adjustments to living with unrelated person(s) (e.g., roommate)

_____ 31. Lower evaluation of your work than you hoped for

_____ 32. Conflicts with family member(s)

_____ 33. Finding your work too demanding

_____ 34. Conflicts with friend(s)

_____ 35. Hard effort to get ahead

_____ 36. Trying to secure loan(s)

_____ 37. Getting "ripped off" or cheated in the purchase of goods

_____ 38. Dissatisfaction with your ability at written expression

_____ 39. Unwanted interruptions of your work

_____ 40. Social isolation

_____ 41. Being ignored

_____ 42. Dissatisfaction with your physical appearance

_____ 43. Unsatisfactory housing conditions

_____ 44. Finding work uninteresting

_____ 45. Failing to get money you expected

_____ 46. Gossip about someone you care about

_____ 47. Dissatisfaction with your physical fitness

_____ 48. Gossip about yourself

_____ 49. Difficulty dealing with modern technology (e.g., computers)

_____ 50. Car problems

_____ 51. Hard work to look after and maintain home

Scoring
Add up your responses and find your rating below.

Very high stress	≥ 136
High stress	116–135
Average stress	76–115
Low stress	56–75
Very low stress	51–55

QUIZ SOURCE: Used with permission from Kohn, P. M., and J. E. Macdonald. 1992. The survey of recent life experiences: A decontaminated hassles scale for adults. *Journal of Behavioral Medicine* 15: 221–236.

Name _____ Section _____ Date _____

WELLNESS WORKSHEET 10

Are You a Type A or a Type B?

You can get a general idea of which personality type you more closely resemble by responding to the following statements. Read each statement and circle one of the numbers that follow it, depending on whether the statement is definitely true for you, mostly true, mostly false, or definitely false. Scoring is explained below.

1 = definitely true   2 = mostly true   3 = mostly false   4 = definitely false

1. I am more restless and fidgety than most people.	1	2	3	4
2. In comparison with most people I know, I'm not very involved in my work.	1	2	3	4
3. I ordinarily work quickly and energetically.	1	2	3	4
4. I rarely have trouble finishing my work.	1	2	3	4
5. I hate giving up before I'm absolutely sure I'm licked.	1	2	3	4
6. I am rather deliberate in telephone conversations.	1	2	3	4
7. I am often in a hurry.	1	2	3	4
8. I am somewhat relaxed and at ease about my work.	1	2	3	4
9. My achievements are considered to be significantly higher than those of most people I know.	1	2	3	4
10. Tailgating bothers me more than a car in front slowing me up.	1	2	3	4
11. In conversation I often gesture with hands and head.	1	2	3	4
12. I rarely drive a car too fast.	1	2	3	4
13. I prefer work in which I can move around.	1	2	3	4
14. People consider me to be rather quiet.	1	2	3	4
15. Sometimes I think I shouldn't work so hard, but something drives me on.	1	2	3	4
16. I usually speak more softly than most people.	1	2	3	4
17. My handwriting is rather fast.	1	2	3	4
18. I often work slowly and deliberately.	1	2	3	4
19. I thrive on challenging situations. The more challenges I have the better.	1	2	3	4
20. I prefer to linger over a meal and enjoy it.	1	2	3	4
21. I like to drive a car rather fast when there is no speed limit.	1	2	3	4
22. I like work that is not too challenging.	1	2	3	4
23. In general I approach my work more seriously than most people I know.	1	2	3	4
24. I talk more slowly than most people.	1	2	3	4
25. I've often been asked to be an officer of some group or groups.	1	2	3	4
26. I often let a problem work itself out by waiting.	1	2	3	4
27. I often try to persuade others to my point of view.	1	2	3	4

(over)

Insel/Roth, *Core Concepts in Health*, Eighth Edition. © 1998 Mayfield Publishing Company. Chapter 2
Insel et al., *Core Concepts in Health*, Brief Eighth Edition. © 1998 Mayfield Publishing Company. Chapter 2

28. I generally walk more slowly than most people.	1	2	3	4
29. I eat rapidly even when there is plenty of time.	1	2	3	4
30. I usually work fast.	1	2	3	4
31. I get very impatient when I'm behind a slow driver and can't pass.	1	2	3	4
32. It makes me mad when I see people not living up to their potential.	1	2	3	4
33. I enjoy being around children.	1	2	3	4
34. I prefer walking to jogging.	1	2	3	4
35. When I'm in the express line at the supermarket, I count the number of items the person ahead of me has and comment if it's over the limit.	1	2	3	4
36. I enjoy reading for pleasure.	1	2	3	4
37. I have high standards for myself and others.	1	2	3	4
38. I like hanging around talking to my friends.	1	2	3	4
39. I often feel that others are taking advantage of me or being inconsiderate.	1	2	3	4
40. If someone is in a hurry, I don't mind letting him or her go ahead of me.	1	2	3	4

Scoring

For each statement, two numbers represent Type A answers and two numbers represent Type B answers. Use the scoring sheet to determine how many Type A and Type B answers you gave. For example, if you circled 1, definitely true, for the first statement, you chose a Type A answer. Add up all your Type A answers and give yourself plus 1 point for each of them. Add up all your Type B answers and give yourself minus 1 point for them.

1. 1,2 = A; 3,4 = B	11. 1,2 = A; 3,4 = B	21. 1,2 = A; 3,4 = B	31. 1,2 = A; 3,4 = B
2. 1,2 = B; 3,4 = A	12. 1,2 = B; 3,4 = A	22. 1,2 = B; 3,4 = A	32. 1,2 = A; 3,4 = B
3. 1,2 = A; 3,4 = B	13. 1,2 = A; 3,4 = B	23. 1,2 = A; 3,4 = B	33. 1,2 = B; 3,4 = A
4. 1,2 = B; 3,4 = A	14. 1,2 = B; 3,4 = A	24. 1,2 = B; 3,4 = A	34. 1,2 = B; 3,4 = A
5. 1,2 = A; 3,4 = B	15. 1,2 = A; 3,4 = B	25. 1,2 = A; 3,4 = B	35. 1,2 = A; 3,4 = B
6. 1,2 = B; 3,4 = A	16. 1,2 = B; 3,4 = A	26. 1,2 = B; 3,4 = A	36. 1,2 = B; 3,4 = A
7. 1,2 = A; 3,4 = B	17. 1,2 = A; 3,4 = B	27. 1,2 = A; 3,4 = B	37. 1,2 = A; 3,4 = B
8. 1,2 = B; 3,4 = A	18. 1,2 = B; 3,4 = A	28. 1,2 = B; 3,4 = A	38. 1,2 = B; 3,4 = A
9. 1,2 = A; 3,4 = B	19. 1,2 = A; 3,4 = B	29. 1,2 = A; 3,4 = B	39. 1,2 = A; 3,4 = B
10. 1,2 = B; 3,4 = A	20. 1,2 = B; 3,4 = A	30. 1,2 = A; 3,4 = B	40. 1,2 = B; 3,4 = A

Total number of Type A answers: _____ × 1 point each = _____
Total number of Type B answers: _____ × −1 point each = _____
Total score (add lines above_____

Determine your personality type based on your total score:
+20 to + 40 = Definite A
 +1 to + 19 = Moderate A
  0 to −19 = Moderate B
−20 to −40 = Definite B

Name _____ Section _____ Date _____

WELLNESS WORKSHEET 11

Social Support

Part I. Assessing Your Level of Social Support

To determine whether your social network measures up, check whether each of the following statements is true or false for you.

True   **False**

_____ _____   1. If I needed an emergency loan of $100, there is someone I could get it from.

_____ _____   2. There is someone who takes pride in my accomplishments.

_____ _____   3. I often meet or talk with family or friends.

_____ _____   4. Most people I know think highly of me.

_____ _____   5. If I needed an early morning ride to the airport, there's no one I would feel comfortable asking to take me.

_____ _____   6. I feel there is no one with whom I can share my most private worries and fears.

_____ _____   7. Most of my friends are more successful making changes in their lives than I am.

_____ _____   8. I would have a hard time finding someone to go with me on a day trip to the beach or country.

Scoring

Add up the number of true answers to questions 1–4 and the number of false answers to questions 5–8. If your score is 4 or more, you should have enough support to protect your health. If your score is 3 or less, refer to your textbook for suggestions on how to build up your social network.

Part II. Social Support Profile

Learn more about your network of social support by completing a social support profile. For each type of support listed below, check or list the people who most often provide that type of support for you. Put an asterisk in the box if that person reciprocates by coming to you for the same type of support.

TYPE OF SUPPORT	**Emotional** Someone you can trust with your most intimate thoughts and fears	**Social** Someone with whom you can hang out and share life experiences	**Informational** Someone you can ask for advice on major decisions	**Practical** Someone who will help you out in a pinch
Partner				
Relative				
Friend				
Neighbor				
Coworker or boss				
Therapist or minister				

(over)

Insel/Roth, *Core Concepts in Health,* Eighth Edition. © 1998 Mayfield Publishing Company. Chapter 2

Insel et al., *Core Concepts in Health,* Brief Eighth Edition. © 1998 Mayfield Publishing Company. Chapter 2

INTERNET ACTIVITY

The Internet can be a valuable resource for building up your social support network. Think about your hobbies and areas of interest. With the Internet, you can get in touch with organizations and people who share your interests. For example, from Yahoo's recreation and sports listings (http://www.yahoo.com_ Recreation), roller bladers can learn about equipment and technique as well as local clubs and skating events. If you are interested in human rights, Amnesty International's home page can put you in touch with a local chapter of the organization. Whatever your interests, odds are that you can find applicable Web pages, bulletin boards, chat rooms, and other Internet resources.

Choose a topic, and use a search engine to locate online resources. Describe what you find: What sites are available? What sorts of information can you obtain? Are there opportunities for you to interact online with people who share your area of interest? Did you find any organizations or groups operating in your area?

Area of interest:_____

Resources located:

QUIZ SOURCE: Japenga, A. 1995. A family of friends. *Health,* November/December. SUPPORT PROFILE SOURCE: Adapted from How supportive is your social circle? 1997. *Health,* April.

Name _____ Section _____ Date _____

WELLNESS WORKSHEET 12

Problem Solving

Do you frequently increase your stress level by stewing over problems, small and large? You can generate an action plan in just a few minutes by going through a formal process of problem solving.

State the problem in one or two sentences:

Identify the key causes of the problem:

List three possible solutions:

1. _____

2. _____

3. _____

List the consequences, good and bad, of each solution:

1. _____

   _____

2. _____

   _____

3. _____

   _____

(over)

Insel/Roth, *Core Concepts in Health,* Eighth Edition. © 1998 Mayfield Publishing Company. Chapter 2
Insel et al., *Core Concepts in Health,* Brief Eighth Edition. © 1998 Mayfield Publishing Company. Chapter 2

Choose the solution that you think will work best for you:

Make a list of what you will need to do to carry out your decision. Designate a time for doing each item on your list.

After you have tried your solution, evaluate it. Was it entirely successful? What will you try differently next time?

WELLNESS WORKSHEET 13

Maslow's Characteristics of a Self-Actualized Person

In the spaces given below, describe yourself in relation to each of Maslow's characteristics of a self-actualized person. How closely does the description fit you? Where would you like to make changes?

1. **Clear perception of reality and comfortable relations with it.** The self-actualized person judges others accurately and is capable of tolerating uncertainty and ambiguity.

2. **Acceptance of self and others.** Self-actualizers accept themselves as they are and are not defensive. They have little guilt, shame, or anxiety.

3. **Natural and spontaneous.** Self-actualizers are spontaneous in both thought and behavior.

4. **Focus on problems rather than self.** Self-actualizers focus on problems outside themselves; they are concerned with basic issues and eternal questions.

5. **Need privacy; tend to be detached.** Although self-actualizers enjoy others, they do not mind solitude and sometimes seek it.

6. **Autonomous.** Self-actualizers are relatively independent of their culture and environment, but they do not go against convention just for the sake of being different.

7. **Continued freshness of appreciation.** Self-actualizers are capable of fresh, spontaneous, and nonstereo-typed appreciation of objects, events, and people. They appreciate the basic pleasures of life.

(over)

Insel/Roth, *Core Concepts in Health,* Eighth Edition. © 1998 Mayfield Publishing Company. Chapter 3
Insel et al., *Core Concepts in Health,* Brief Eighth Edition. © 1998 Mayfield Publishing Company. Chapter 3

8. **Mystic experience.** Self-actualizers have had peak experiences or experiences in which they have attained transcendence.

9. **Social interest.** Self-actualizers have feelings of identification, sympathy, and affection for others.

10. **Interpersonal relations.** Self-actualizers do on occasion get angry, but they do not bear long-lasting grudges. Their relationships with others are few but are deep and meaningful.

11. **Democratic character structure.** Self-actualizers show respect for all people irrespective of race, creed, income level, etc.

12. **Discrimination between means and ends.** Self-actualizers are strongly ethical with definite moral standards. They do not confuse means with ends; they relate to ends rather than means.

13. **Sense of humor.** Self-actualizers have a sense of humor that is both philosophical and nonhostile.

14. **Creativeness.** Self-actualizers are original and inventive, expressive, perceptive, and spontaneous in everyday life. They are able to see things in new ways.

15. **Nonconformity.** Self-actualizers fit into their culture, but they are independent of it and do not blindly comply with all its demands. They are open to new experiences.

WELLNESS WORKSHEET 14

Personal Identity and Values

Developing a personal identity and a guiding set of values or beliefs are key tasks of adulthood. Take a few minutes now to examine your identity and values.

Part I. Identity

Make a list of the characteristics, attitudes, beliefs, interests, activities, and relationships that make up your personal identity. What adjectives best describe you? Circle the five that you think are most important to your self-concept.

What are your strong and weak points? List at least five of each.

What do you think of as your key accomplishments to date?

What are your major goals for the future? How do you picture yourself in 10 years?

(over)

Insel/Roth, *Core Concepts in Health,* Eighth Edition. © 1998 Mayfield Publishing Company. Chapter 3
Insel et al., *Core Concepts in Health,* Brief Eighth Edition. © 1998 Mayfield Publishing Company. Chapter 3

Part II. Values

List the personality traits or characteristics that you most value—e.g., friendly, patient, successful, outgoing, cooperative, loyal to family and friends. These can be characteristics of your own or of others.

List the activities or accomplishments that you most value—e.g., making lots of money, getting good grades, spending time with friends, making one's own decisions. These can be accomplishments of your own or of others or goals you have for the future.

List the social ideals, customs, and institutions that you value—e.g., education, equality, freedom of speech, tolerance for diverse opinions.

How do your values compare with your personal identity and goals?

WELLNESS WORKSHEET 15

The General Well-Being Scale

For each question, choose the answer that best describes how you have felt and how things have been going for you *during the past month*.

1. How have you been feeling in general?

   5 _____ In excellent spirits

   4 _____ In very good spirits

   3 _____ In good spirits mostly

   2 _____ I've been up and down in spirits a lot

   1 _____ In low spirits mostly

   0 _____ In very low spirits

2. Have you been bothered by nervousness or your "nerves"?

   0 _____ Extremely so—to the point where I could not work or take care of things

   1 _____ Very much so

   2 _____ Quite a bit

   3 _____ Some—enough to bother me

   4 _____ A little

   5 _____ Not at all

3. Have you been in firm control of your behavior, thoughts, emotions or feelings?

   5 _____ Yes, definitely so

   4 _____ Yes, for the most part

   3 _____ Generally so

   2 _____ Not too well

   1 _____ No, and I am somewhat disturbed

   0 _____ No, and I am very disturbed

4. Have you felt so sad, discouraged, hopeless, or had so many problems that you wondered if anything was worthwhile?

   0 _____ Extremely so—to the point I have just about given up

   1 _____ Very much so

   2 _____ Quite a bit

   3 _____ Some—enough to bother me

   4 _____ A little bit

   5 _____ Not at all

(over)

Insel/Roth, *Core Concepts in Health,* Eighth Edition. © 1998 Mayfield Publishing Company. Chapter 3

Insel et al., *Core Concepts in Health,* Brief Eighth Edition. © 1998 Mayfield Publishing Company. Chapter 3

5. Have you been under or felt you were under any strain, stress, or pressure?

    0 _____ Yes—almost more than I could bear

    1 _____ Yes—quite a bit of pressure

    2 _____ Yes—some, more than usual

    3 _____ Yes—some, but about usual

    4 _____ Yes—a little

    5 _____ Not at all

6. How happy, satisfied, or pleased have you been with your personal life?

    5 _____ Extremely happy—couldn't have been more satisfied or pleased

    4 _____ Very happy

    3 _____ Fairly happy

    2 _____ Satisfied—pleased

    1 _____ Somewhat dissatisfied

    0 _____ Very dissatisfied

7. Have you had reason to wonder if you were losing your mind, or losing control over the way you act, talk, think, feel, or of your memory?

    5 _____ Not at all

    4 _____ Only a little

    3 _____ Some, but not enough to be concerned

    2 _____ Some, and I've been a little concerned

    1 _____ Some, and I am quite concerned

    0 _____ Much, and I'm very concerned

8. Have you been anxious, worried, or upset?

    0 _____ Extremely so—to the point of being sick, or almost sick

    1 _____ Very much so

    2 _____ Quite a bit

    3 _____ Some—enough to bother me

    4 _____ A little bit

    5 _____ Not at all

9. Have you been waking up fresh and rested?

    5 _____ Every day

    4 _____ Most every day

    3 _____ Fairly often

    2 _____ Less than half the time

    1 _____ Rarely

    0 _____ None of the time

(over)

10. Have you been bothered by any illness, bodily disorder, pain, or fears about your health?

    0 _____ All the time

    1 _____ Most of the time

    2 _____ A good bit of the time

    3 _____ Some of the time

    4 _____ A little of the time

    5 _____ None of the time

11. Has your daily life been full of things that are interesting to you?

    5 _____ All the time

    4 _____ Most of the time

    3 _____ A good bit of the time

    2 _____ Some of the time

    1 _____ A little of the time

    0 _____ None of the time

12. Have you felt downhearted and blue?

    0 _____ All of the time

    1 _____ Most of the time

    2 _____ A good bit of the time

    3 _____ Some of the time

    4 _____ A little of the time

    5 _____ None of the time

13. Have you been feeling emotionally stable and sure of yourself?

    5 _____ All of the time

    4 _____ Most of the time

    3 _____ A good bit of the time

    2 _____ Some of the time

    1 _____ A little of the time

    0 _____ None of the time

14. Have you felt tired, worn out, used-up, or exhausted?

    0 _____ All of the time

    1 _____ Most of the time

    2 _____ A good bit of the time

    3 _____ Some of the time

    4 _____ A little of the time

    5 _____ None of the time

(over)

Circle the number that seems closest to how you have felt generally *during the past month.*

15. How concerned or worried about your health have you been?

Not concerned at all	10	8	6	4	2	0	**Very concerned**

16. How relaxed or tense have you been?

Very relaxed	10	8	6	4	2	0	**Very tense**

17. How much energy, pep, and vitality have you felt?

No energy at all, listless	0	2	4	6	8	10	**Very energetic, dynamic**

18. How depressed or cheerful have you been?

Very depressed	0	2	4	6	8	10	**Very cheerful**

Scoring
Add up all the points for the answers you have chosen, and find your score below.

81–110	Positive well-being
76–80	Low positive
71–75	Marginal
56–70	Stress problem
41–55	Distress
26–40	Serious
0–25	Severe

SOURCE: National Center for Health Statistics. General Well-Being Scale (GWBS).

WELLNESS WORKSHEET 16

Self-Esteem Inventory

Read each of the following statements; check the "like me" column if it describes how you usually feel and the "unlike me" column if it does not describe how you usually feel.

Like me   Unlike me

_____   _____   1. I spend a lot of time daydreaming.

_____   _____   2. I'm pretty sure of myself.

_____   _____   3. I often wish I were someone else.

_____   _____   4. I'm easy to like.

_____   _____   5. My family and I have a lot of fun together.

_____   _____   6. I never worry about anything.

_____   _____   7. I find it very hard to talk in front of a group.

_____   _____   8. I wish I were younger.

_____   _____   9. There are lots of things about myself I'd change if I could.

_____   _____   10. I can make up my mind without too much trouble.

_____   _____   11. I'm a lot of fun to be with.

_____   _____   12. I get upset easily at home.

_____   _____   13. I always do the right thing.

_____   _____   14. I'm proud of my work.

_____   _____   15. Someone always has to tell me what to do.

_____   _____   16. It takes me a long time to get used to anything new.

_____   _____   17. I'm often sorry for the things I do.

_____   _____   18. I'm popular with people my own age.

_____   _____   19. My family usually considers my feelings.

_____   _____   20. I'm never happy.

_____   _____   21. I'm doing the best work that I can.

(over)

Like me   Unlike me

_____   _____   22. I give in very easily.

_____   _____   23. I can usually take care of myself.

_____   _____   24. I'm pretty happy.

_____   _____   25. I would rather associate with people younger than me.

_____   _____   26. My family expects too much of me.

_____   _____   27. I like everyone I know.

_____   _____   28. I like to be called on when I am in a group.

_____   _____   29. I understand myself.

_____   _____   30. It's pretty tough to be me.

_____   _____   31. Things are all mixed up in my life.

_____   _____   32. People usually follow my ideas.

_____   _____   33. No one pays much attention to me at home.

_____   _____   34. I never get scolded.

_____   _____   35. I'm not doing as well at work as I'd like to.

_____   _____   36. I can make up my mind and stick to it.

_____   _____   37. I really don't like being a man/woman.

_____   _____   38. I have a low opinion of myself.

_____   _____   39. I don't like to be with other people.

_____   _____   40. There are many times when I'd like to leave home.

_____   _____   41. I'm never shy.

_____   _____   42. I often feel upset.

_____   _____   43. I often feel ashamed of myself.

_____   _____   44. I'm not as nice-looking as most people.

_____   _____   45. If I have something to say, I usually say it.

(over)

Like me   Unlike me

_____   _____   46. People pick on me very often.

_____   _____   47. My family understands me.

_____   _____   48. I always tell the truth.

_____   _____   49. My employer or supervisor makes me feel I'm not good enough.

_____   _____   50. I don't care what happens to me.

_____   _____   51. I'm a failure.

_____   _____   52. I get upset easily when I am scolded.

_____   _____   53. Most people are better liked than I am.

_____   _____   54. I usually feel as if my family is pushing me.

_____   _____   55. I always know what to say to people.

_____   _____   56. I often get discouraged.

_____   _____   57. Things usually don't bother me.

_____   _____   58. I can't be depended on.

Scoring
The test has a built in "lie scale" to help determine if you are trying too hard to appear to have high self-esteem. If you answered "like me" to three or more of the following items, retake the test with an eye toward being more realistic in your responses: 1, 6, 13, 20, 27, 34, 41, 48.

To calculate your score, add up the number of times your responses match those given below. To determine how your level of self-esteem compares to that of others, find the value closest to your score in the appropriate column of the table.

     Like me: Items 2, 4, 5, 10, 11, 14, 18, 19, 21, 23, 24, 28, 29, 32, 36, 45, 47, 55, 57
  Unlike me: Items 3, 7, 8, 9, 12, 15, 16, 17, 22, 25, 26, 30, 31, 33, 35, 37, 38, 39, 40, 42, 43, 44, 46, 49,
                50, 51, 52, 53, 54, 56, 58

Men	Women	
33	32	Significantly below average
36	35	Somewhat below average
40	39	Average
44	43	Somewhat above average
47	46	Significantly above average

SOURCE: Adapted and reproduced with permission of author and publisher from Ryden, M. B. 1978. An adult version of the Coopersmith Self-Esteem Inventory: Test-retest reliability and social desirability. *Psychological Reports* 43: 1189–1190. © 1978 Psychological Reports.

Name _____ Section _____ Date _____

WELLNESS WORKSHEET 17

How Assertive Are You?

For each statement, indicate how characteristic or descriptive it is for you by writing in the appropriate number.

+3 = very characteristic of me, extremely descriptive
+2 = rather characteristic of me, quite descriptive
+1 = somewhat characteristic of me, slightly descriptive
−1 = somewhat uncharacteristic of me, slightly nondescriptive
−2 = rather uncharacteristic of me, quite nondescriptive
−3 = very uncharacteristic of me, extremely nondescriptive

_____ 1. Most people seem to be more aggressive and assertive than I am.

_____ 2. I have hesitated to make or accept dates because of shyness.

_____ 3. When the food served at a restaurant is not done to my satisfaction, I complain about it to the waiter or waitress.

_____ 4. I am careful to avoid hurting other peoples' feelings, even when I feel that I have been injured.

_____ 5. If a salesperson has gone to considerable trouble to show me merchandise that is not quite suitable, I have a difficult time saying no.

_____ 6. When I am asked to do something, I insist upon knowing why.

_____ 7. There are times when I look for a good, vigorous argument.

_____ 8. I strive to get ahead as well as most people in my position.

_____ 9. To be honest, people often take advantage of me.

_____ 10. I enjoy starting conversations with new acquaintances and strangers.

_____ 11. I often don't know what to say to attractive persons of the opposite sex.

_____ 12. I hesitate to make phone calls to business establishments and institutions.

_____ 13. I would rather apply for a job or for admission to a college by writing letters than by going through with personal interviews.

_____ 14. I find it embarrassing to return merchandise.

_____ 15. If a close and respected relative were annoying me, I would smother my feelings rather than express my annoyance.

_____ 16. I have avoided asking questions for fear of sounding stupid.

_____ 17. During an argument I am sometimes afraid that I will get so upset that I will shake all over.

_____ 18. If a famed and respected lecturer makes a statement that I think is incorrect, I will have the audience hear my point of view as well.

_____ 19. I avoid arguing over prices with clerks and salesmen.

(over)

Insel/Roth, *Core Concepts in Health,* Eighth Edition. © 1998 Mayfield Publishing Company. Chapter 3
Insel et al., *Core Concepts in Health,* Brief Eighth Edition. © 1998 Mayfield Publishing Company. Chapter 3

_____ 20. When I have done something important or worthwhile, I manage to let others know about it.

_____ 21. I am open and frank about my feelings.

_____ 22. If someone has been spreading false and bad stories about me, I see that person as soon as possible to have a talk about it.

_____ 23. I often have a hard time saying no.

_____ 24. I tend to bottle up my emotions rather than make a scene.

_____ 25. I complain about poor service in a restaurant or elsewhere.

_____ 26. When I am given a compliment, I sometimes just don't know what to say.

_____ 27. If a couple near me in a theater or at a lecture were conversing rather loudly, I would ask them to be quiet or to take their conversation elsewhere.

_____ 28. Anyone attempting to push ahead of me in a line is in for a good battle.

_____ 29. I am quick to express an opinion.

_____ 30. There are times when I just can't say anything.

Scoring

Some of the items in this test are reverse scored, so you need to change the sign of your answer. For the items listed below, if you answered with a negative number, change the sign from a minus to a plus; if you answered with a positive number, change the sign from a plus to a minus.

1	5	12	15	19	26
2	9	13	16	23	30
4	11	14	17	24	

Next, total your scores, and find your rating below. (You may find it easier to add up your positive and negative scores separately and then subtract the total of your negative scores from the total of your positive scores.)

–29	Significantly below average
–15	Somewhat below average
0	Average
+15	Somewhat above average
+29	Significantly above average

SOURCE: Rathus, S. A. 1973. A 30-item schedule for assessing assertive behavior. *Behavior Therapy* 4: 398–406. Used by permission.

WELLNESS WORKSHEET 18

How Comfortable Are You in Social Situations?

The statements below are things you may have thought to yourself at some time before, during, or after a social interaction with someone you would like to get to know. Decide how frequently you might have been thinking a similar thought, and enter the appropriate number from the scale below. Please answer as honestly as possible.

1 = hardly ever had the thought
2 = rarely had the thought
3 = sometimes had the thought
4 = often had the thought
5 = very often had the thought

_____ 1. When I can't think of anything to say, I can feel myself getting very anxious.

_____ 2. I can usually talk to women/men pretty well.

_____ 3. I hope I don't make a fool of myself.

_____ 4. I'm beginning to feel more at ease.

_____ 5. I'm really afraid of what she'll/he'll think of me.

_____ 6. No worries, no fears, no anxieties.

_____ 7. I'm scared to death.

_____ 8. She/He probably won't be interested in me.

_____ 9. Maybe I can put her/him at ease by starting things going.

_____ 10. Instead of worrying, I can figure out how best to get to know her/him.

_____ 11. I'm not too comfortable meeting women/men, so things are bound to go wrong.

_____ 12. What the heck, the worst that can happen is that she/he won't go for me.

_____ 13. She/He may want to talk to me as much as I want to talk to her/him.

_____ 14. This will be a good opportunity.

_____ 15. If I blow this conversation, I'll really lose my confidence.

_____ 16. What I say will probably sound stupid.

_____ 17. What do I have to lose? It's worth a try.

_____ 18. This is an awkward situation, but I can handle it.

_____ 19. Wow—I don't want to do this.

_____ 20. It would crush me if she/he didn't respond to me.

_____ 21. I've just got to make a good impression on her/him, or I'll feel terrible.

_____ 22. You're such an inhibited idiot.

_____ 23. I'll probably bomb out anyway.

(over)

Insel/Roth, *Core Concepts in Health,* Eighth Edition. © 1998 Mayfield Publishing Company. Chapter 3
Insel et al., *Core Concepts in Health,* Brief Eighth Edition. © 1998 Mayfield Publishing Company. Chapter 3

_____ 24. I can handle anything.

_____ 25. Even if things don't go well, it's no catastrophe.

_____ 26. I feel awkward and dumb; she's/he's bound to notice.

_____ 27. We probably have a lot in common.

_____ 28. Maybe we'll hit it off real well.

_____ 29. I wish I could leave and avoid the whole situation.

_____ 30. Ah! Throw caution to the wind.

Scoring

For the Positive Thoughts scale, add up your responses to the following questions:

2	4	6	9	10	12	13	14
17	18	24	25	27	28	30	

For the Negative Thoughts scale, add up your responses to the following questions:

1	3	5	7	8	11	15	16
19	20	21	22	23	26	29	

Find your scores on the table below. A high score on the Positive Thoughts scale indicates a high degree of comfort in social situations and a low degree of social anxiety. A high score on the Negative Thoughts scale indicates a high degree of social anxiety. For tips on overcoming social anxiety, refer to the Behavior Change Strategy in Chapter 3 of your text.

Positive Thoughts		Negative Thoughts		
Men	Women	Men	Women	
40	45	34	31	Significantly below average
43	48	39	34	Somewhat below average
47	52	44	38	Average
51	56	49	42	Somewhat above average
54	59	54	45	Significantly above average

SOURCE: Used with permission from Glass, C. R., et al. 1982. The social interaction self-statement test. *Cognitive Therapy and Research*, 37–55.

Name _____ Section _____ Date _____

 WELLNESS WORKSHEET 19

Recognizing Signs of Depression

Part I. Are You Depressed?
Circle the answer that best describes how you have felt over the last week. If you can't decide between two numbers for an item, choose the higher.

	Rarely or none of the time (less than 1 day)	Some or a little of the time (1–2 days)	Occasionally or a moderate amount of the time (3–4 days)	Most or all of the time (5–7 days)
1. I was bothered by things that usually don't bother me.	0	1	2	3
2. I did not feel like eating; my appetite was poor.	0	1	2	3
3. I felt I could not shake off the blues even with help from my family or friends.	0	1	2	3
4. I felt I was just as good as other people.	3	2	1	0
5. I had trouble keeping my mind on what I was doing.	0	1	2	3
6. I felt depressed.	0	1	2	3
7. I felt that everything I did was an effort.	0	1	2	3
8. I felt hopeful about the future.	3	2	1	0
9. I thought my life had been a failure.	0	1	2	3
10. I felt fearful.	0	1	2	3
11. My sleep was restless.	0	1	2	3
12. I was happy.	3	2	1	0
13. I talked less than usual.	0	1	2	3
14. I felt lonely.	0	1	2	3
15. People were unfriendly.	0	1	2	3
16. I enjoyed life.	3	2	1	0
17. I had crying spells.	0	1	2	3
18. I felt sad.	0	1	2	3
19. I felt that people disliked me.	0	1	2	3
20. I could not get going.	0	1	2	3

Scoring
Add up the numbers you circled, and refer to the following list:

Less than 10	Not depressed
10–15	Mild depression
16–24	Moderate depression
Greater than 24	Severe depression

Although occasional mild to moderate symptoms of depression may be normal and not require treatment, more persistent or severe symptoms, especially if accompanied by thoughts of suicide, are a reason to see a mental health professional right away. Don't depend too heavily on any one measure of depression, however. The subjective experience of depression is highly variable. Some people with few subjective symptoms and normal scores on a depression questionnaire are actually quite depressed and respond markedly to treatment.

(over)

Insel/Roth, *Core Concepts in Health*, Eighth Edition. © 1998 Mayfield Publishing Company. Chapter 3
Insel et al., *Core Concepts in Health*, Brief Eighth Edition. © 1998 Mayfield Publishing Company. Chapter 3

Part II. Is a Friend Depressed?

The following are signals that a friend may be depressed. Check any symptom that you have noticed that has persisted longer than 2 weeks.

Does he or she express feelings of

_____ Sadness or "emptiness"?

_____ Hopelessness, pessimism, or guilt?

_____ Helplessness or worthlessness?

Does he or she seem

_____ Unable to make decisions?

_____ Unable to concentrate and remember?

_____ To have lost interest or pleasure in ordinary activities like sports or band or talking on the phone?

_____ To have more problems with school and family?

Does he or she complain of

_____ Loss of energy and drive so they seem "slowed down"?

_____ Trouble falling asleep, staying asleep, or getting up?

_____ Appetite problems—are they losing or gaining weight?

_____ Headaches, stomachaches, or backaches?

_____ Chronic aches and pains in joints and muscles?

Has his or her behavior changed suddenly so that

_____ They are restless or more irritable?

_____ They want to be alone most of the time?

_____ They've started cutting classes or dropped hobbies and activities?

_____ You think they may be drinking heavily or taking drugs?

Has he or she talked about

_____ Death?

_____ Suicide—or attempted suicide?

INTERNET ACTIVITY

Use the Internet to learn more about depression—its causes, symptoms, risks, and treatment. Visit one of the following sites, or do a search to locate a different depression-related site.

American Psychiatric Association: http://www.psych.org

National Institute of Mental Health: http://www.nimh.nih.gov/home.htm

American Psychological Association: http://www.apa.org

National Depressive and Manic-Depressive Association: http://www.ndmda.org

Visit at least one site; describe the resources and information available about depression.

URL:_____

Description of site/information available:

What was the most surprising fact about depression that you learned from the site?

PART I QUIZ SOURCE: Radloff, L. S. 1979. The CES-D scale: A self-report depression scale for research in the general population. *Applied Psychological Measurement* 1: 387. Copyright ©1979 Sage Publications, Inc. Reprinted by permission of the publisher. PART II QUIZ SOURCE: U.S. Department of Health and Human Services. What to do when a friend is depressed, guide for students.

Name _____ Section _____ Date _____

WELLNESS WORKSHEET 20

How Capable Are You of Being Intimate?

Determine how closely each statement describes your feelings. Circle the number in the appropriate column.

	Strongly disagree	Mildly disagree	Agree and disagree equally	Mildly agree	Strongly agree
1. I like to share my feelings with others.	1	2	3	4	5
2. I like to feel close to other people.	1	2	3	4	5
3. I like to listen to other people talk about their feelings.	1	2	3	4	5
4. I am concerned with rejection in my expression of feelings to others.	5	4	3	2	1
5. I'm concerned with being dominated in a close relationship with another.	5	4	3	2	1
6. I'm often anxious about my own acceptance in a close relationship.	5	4	3	2	1
7. I'm concerned that I trust other people too much.	5	4	3	2	1
8. Expression of emotion makes me feel close to another person.	1	2	3	4	5
9. I do not want to express feelings that would hurt another person.	5	4	3	2	1
10. I am overly critical of people in a close relationship.	5	4	3	2	1
11. I want to feel close to people to whom I am attracted.	1	2	3	4	5
12. I tend to reveal my deepest feelings to other people.	1	2	3	4	5
13. I'm afraid to talk about my sexual feelings with a person in whom I'm very interested.	5	4	3	2	1
14. I want to be close to a person who is attracted to me.	1	2	3	4	5
15. I would not become too close because it involves conflict.	5	4	3	2	1
16. I seek out close relationships with people to whom I am attracted.	1	2	3	4	5

(over)

	Strongly disagree	Mildly disagree	Agree and disagree equally	Mildly agree	Strongly agree
17. When people become close they tend not to listen to each other.	5	4	3	2	1
18. Intimate relationships bring me great satisfaction.	1	2	3	4	5
19. I search for close intimate relationships.	1	2	3	4	5
20. It is important to me to form close relationships.	1	2	3	4	5
21. I do not need to share my feelings and thoughts with others.	5	4	3	2	1
22. When I become very close to another, I am likely to see things that are hard for me to accept.	5	4	3	2	1
23. I tend to accept most things about people with whom I share a close relationship.	1	2	3	4	5
24. I defend my personal space so others do not come too close.	5	4	3	2	1
25. I tend to distrust people who are concerned with closeness and intimacy.	5	4	3	2	1
26. I have concerns about losing my individuality in close relationships.	5	4	3	2	1
27. I have concerns about giving up control if I enter into a really intimate relationship.	5	4	3	2	1
28. Being honest and open with another person makes me feel closer to that person.	1	2	3	4	5
29. If I were another person, I would be interested in getting to know me.	1	2	3	4	5
30. I only become close to people with whom I share common interests.	5	4	3	2	1
31. Revealing secrets about my sex life makes me feel close to others.	1	2	3	4	5
32. Generally, I can feel just as close to someone of the same sex as someone of the other sex.	1	2	3	4	5
33. When another person is physically attracted to me, I usually want to become more intimate.	1	2	3	4	5
34. I have difficulty being intimate with more than one person.	5	4	3	2	1

(over)

	Strongly disagree	Mildly disagree	Agree and disagree equally	Mildly agree	Strongly agree
35. Being open and intimate with another person usually makes me feel good.	1	2	3	4	5
36. I usually can see another person's point of view.	1	2	3	4	5
37. I want to be sure that I am in good control of myself before I attempt to become intimate with another person.	5	4	3	2	1
38. I resist intimacy.	5	4	3	2	1
39. Stories of interpersonal relationships tend to affect me.	1	2	3	4	5
40. Undressing with members of a group increases my feelings of intimacy.	5	4	3	2	1
41. I try to trust and be close to others.	1	2	3	4	5
42. I think that people who want to become intimate have hidden reasons for wanting closeness.	5	4	3	2	1
43. When I become intimate with another person, the possibility of my being manipulated is increased.	5	4	3	2	1
44. I am generally a secretive person.	5	4	3	2	1
45. I feel that sex and intimacy are the same, and one cannot exist without the other.	5	4	3	2	1
46. I can only be intimate in a physical relationship.	5	4	3	2	1
47. The demands placed on me by those with whom I have intimate relationships often inhibit my own satisfaction.	5	4	3	2	1
48. I would compromise to maintain an intimate relationship.	1	2	3	4	5
49. When I am physically attracted to another, I usually want to become intimate with the person.	1	2	3	4	5
50. I understand and accept that intimacy leads to bad feelings as well as good feelings.	1	2	3	4	5

(over)

Scoring

To calculate your total score, add up the items you circled. Find the score below that is closest to your total score.

150	Significantly below average
161	Somewhat below average
172	Average
183	Somewhat above average
194	Significantly above average

SOURCE: Amidon, E., V. K. Kumar, and T. Treadwell. 1983. Measurement of intimacy attitudes: The intimacy attitude scale—revised. *Journal of Personality Assessment*, 635–639. Used by permission.

Name _____ Section _____ Date _____

Part I. How Satisfying Is Your Relationship?

For each item, circle the number that reflects your relationship:

1. How well does your partner meet your needs?	1 Poorly	2	3 Average	4	5 Extremely well
2. In general, how satisfied are you with your relationship?	1 Unsatisfied	2	3 Average	4	5 Extremely satisfied
3. How good is your relationship compared to most?	1 Poor	2	3 Average	4	5 Excellent
4. How often do you wish you hadn't gotten into this relationship?	1 Never	2	3 Average	4	5 Very often
5. To what extent has your relationship met your original expectations?	1 Hardly at all	2	3 Average	4	5 Completely
6. How much do you love your partner?	1 Not much	2	3 Average	4	5 Very much
7. How many problems are there in your relationship?	1 Very few	2	3 Average	4	5 Very many

Add up your points for all seven items, and find the number closest to your total below.

Score	How satisfying is your relationship compared to the average relationship?
23 or below	Substantially less satisfying
26	Moderately less satisfying
29	About as satisfying as average
32	Moderately more satisfying
35 or above	Substantially more satisfying

Part II. How Compatible Are You and Your Prospective Partner?

Both you and your partner should take the quiz below and then compare your answers. This quiz is not meant to be a valid scientific measure of your compatibility; it was put together to get you thinking about situations that can be difficult and cause stress in a relationship. It's perfectly OK to have some disagreement—provided you're able to compromise or, at least, agree to disagree. Suggestions for each of the issues mentioned follow the quiz.

1. How many of the 10 items on this list do you have in common with your prospective mate: religion, career, same hometown or neighborhood, friends, education level, income level, cultural pastimes, sports/recreation activities, travel, physical attraction?

2. Would you prefer a relationship that is
   a. Male-dominated.
   b. Female-dominated.
   c. A partnership.

3. What banking arrangement sounds best after marriage?
   a. Separate accounts.
   b. Joint account.
   c. Joint account but some cash for each of you to spend as you please with no accounting.

(over)

Insel/Roth, *Core Concepts in Health,* Eighth Edition. © 1998 Mayfield Publishing Company. Chapter 4
Insel et al., *Core Concepts in Health,* Brief Eighth Edition. © 1998 Mayfield Publishing Company. Chapter 4

4. If you share an account, whose responsibility should it be to balance the checkbook and pay bills?
   a. The man in the family.
   b. The woman in the family.
   c. Whoever is better at math and details.

5. If you inherited $10,000, would you prefer it to be:
   a. Saved toward a major purchase.
   b. Spent on something you could enjoy together, such as a vacation.
   c. Spent on luxury items you could enjoy individually, such as a fur coat or golf clubs.

6. Where do you think you should spend major holidays?
   a. With his family.
   b. With her family.
   c. Alternating with his and her family.

7. How frequently do you want to see your in-laws if they live in the same town?
   a. Only on special occasions and holidays.
   b. Twice a month.
   c. At least once a week.

8. How frequently do you enjoy talking with your parents?
   a. Every day.
   b. Once a week.
   c. Once a month or less.

9. If you both have careers, what will be your priority?
   a. Marriage before career.
   b. Marriage equally important to career.
   c. Career before marriage; my spouse is going to have to be understanding.

10. If you are offered a career promotion with a hefty raise making your income much more than your spouse's but involving a move out of state, would you
    a. Expect your mate to be agreeable to relocation.
    b. Try a commuter marriage; only seeing each other weekends or occasionally.
    c. Say no rather than move; money isn't everything.

11. If your new spouse sets aside one evening a week to go out with a friend or friends of his or her same sex, would you feel

    a. Jealous of the time away from you.
    b. Happy that he or she has friends.
    c. This should not go on; let your feelings be known.

12. If you've had a bad day at the office and come home feeling moody, would you prefer that your mate
    a. Back off, get out of the way.
    b. Act sympathetic, be a good listener.
    c. Discuss the events that led to your mood, perhaps offering some alternative suggestions for dealing with the people or problems that made you unhappy.

13. If your mate does something that makes you extremely angry, are you most likely to
    a. Forgive and forget it.
    b. Hurl insults.
    c. Mention you are angry at an appropriate time, preferably when the anger is first felt, and explain why without making derogatory accusations.

14. If you can't stand his or her friends and he or she can't stand yours, how will you deal with this after marriage? (You may choose more than one.)
    a. Cultivate new friends that you both can enjoy.
    b. See your friends by yourself; let him or her do the same.
    c. Phase out the friends you knew before marriage; expect your partner to do the same.

15. If you and your spouse-to-be are different religions, would you expect to
    a. Convert before marriage.
    b. Have him or her convert before marriage.
    c. Take turns attending each other's place of worship.
    d. Observe religious days separately.
    e. Not worry about it; religion is not an issue in your relationship.

16. When do you want to start a family?
    a. As soon as possible.
    b. After you have spent a few years enjoying your relationship as a couple.
    c. As soon as careers are firmly established.
    d. Never.

(over)

17. What is your attitude about housework? (You may check more than one.)
    a. It is unmasculine for a man to do it. A woman should do all of it even if she chooses to have a career.
    b. It is fine for a man to help, but only with certain tasks, such as mowing the lawn or taking out the trash.
    c. If a woman works outside the home, cleaning should be shared.
    d. Even if a woman does not work outside the home, cleaning should be shared.

18. Before marriage, you go out as a couple several times a week. A few months after marriage, you realize that you are going out a lot less. Would you consider this
    a. OK. The pace was exhausting.
    b. Dull. You worry that you are being taken for granted.
    c. Not OK. You and your mate should make plans for some evenings out or evenings at home with friends.

19. You need to buy a new suit. Your spouse wants to come along. Would you see this as a sign of
    a. Interest in spending time with you.
    b. Crowding your relationship.
    c. Watch-dogging your taste or pocketbook.

20. How would you prefer to spend your annual vacation? (Choose as many as apply.)
    a. On a trip by yourself.
    b. On a trip with your mate.
    c. On a trip with your mate and another couple.
    d. Visiting your relatives or in-laws at their homes.
    e. At a beach relaxing.
    f. Engaged in an active sport such as skiing, tennis camp, or hiking/camping.
    g. Traveling to another city for sightseeing/shopping.
    h. At home catching up on repairs, appointments, books, visits with friends.
    i. I would rather take a vacation less frequently than once a year and spend this money on rent or mortgage, enabling us to live in a more convenient or prestigious neighborhood.

21. If you were hunting for a place to live, would you prefer being in
    a. The country.
    b. The suburbs.
    c. The city.

22. If your spouse-to-be had many loves before he or she met you, would you prefer that he or she
    a. Keep the details to himself or herself.
    b. Tell you everything.
    c. Answer truthfully but only the questions you ask, such as what broke up each relationship.

23. If your new spouse is in a romantic mood and you are not, how would you be most likely to respond?
    a. Communicate your mood; suggest another time.
    b. Pretend you are feeling romantic.
    c. Invent an excuse rather than communicate your mood.

Once you and your prospective partner have completed the questionnaire, compare your answers with the following commentary in mind.

1. The more you have in common, the more of your life you can share and enjoy together.

2. Research and experiences of many couples have shown that the equal relationship is most successful.

3 and 4. There is not one right answer. Decide what works best for you and creates the least tension in your relationship.

5. You need to understand your priorities and be able to communicate them to your partner. Without this, you can find yourself in great financial conflict and tension.

6. Be able to compromise on this one.

7 and 8. Let your spouse know that he or she comes first before parents and in-laws regardless of how often relatives will be seen.

9. Talk about career and marriage priorities Can you accept your spouse's choice if he or she considers time spent on work more important right now than time spent with you?

(over)

10. There is not one right answer. Decide what works best for you and creates the least tension in your relationship.

11. It's healthy to have friends. You can't realistically expect your mate to spend 24 hours around the clock with you. If you or your mate go off for a time with friends, it wouldn't be too mushy to kiss, hug, or otherwise reassure your mate by words or actions that he or she is still first in your life.

12. There are times when each answer would be best. Be sensitive to your mate's mood. If you are the one in the bad mood, don't expect your mate to read your mind as to whether you need space, sympathy, or discussion. Clue him or her in.

13. Answer C is best. You must learn how to express anger constructively.

14. Be careful here. If you make his or her old friends feel left out or unimportant, they could work on your prospective mate to break up your relationship.

15. If you have major differences on this one, you may want to consider terminating the relationship instead of committing to marriage.

16. It's impossible to have half a child. Compromise won't work on this one, so it is best to speak your mind before marriage.

17. The most successful marriages are the ones in which men and women do not limit themselves in the traditional masculine-feminine roles. The sharing of responsibility/heightens a sense of trust, caring, and cooperation.

18. Sometimes the pace during dating is frantic. It is nice to calm down, but not nice to settle down to the point that each of you is taking the other for granted. Marriage requires continual work if you are going to keep adventure and interest in the relationship.

19. Whether you see it as interest, crowding, or distrust, communicate your feelings to your mate. If you'd rather shop alone, let that be known too.

20. Agree upon your needs in advance of the annual vacation, or what should be a time of relaxation away from the daily grind will turn into a source of tension and arguments. There is nothing wrong with separate vacations if one of you wants to fish on the lake and the other enjoys sightseeing.

21. If you are set on a particular style of living and not willing to change it after marriage, speak up before you say, "I do."

22. In general, it is not a good idea to go into great detail about past relationships because they are not totally relevant to your current one. However, trust and honesty are very important. If your partner asks a question, answer honestly but think very carefully. If you are the one doing the questioning, ask yourself "Do I really want to hear this?"

23. There are times in your relationship when you may not want to go along with your spouse's romantic feelings, but it is generally best to communicate in a nice way without making him or her feel rejected or unloved because you simply are not in the mood. Do suggest another time.

PART I QUIZ SOURCE: Hendrick, S. S. 1988. A generic measure of relationship satisfaction. *Journal of Marriage and the Family* 50: 93–98. Copyright © 1988 by the National Council on Family Relations, 3989 Central Ave., N.E., Ste. 550, Minneapolis, MN 55421. Reprinted by permission.

WELLNESS WORKSHEET 22

Sternberg's Triangular Love Scale

Read each of the following statements, filling in the blank spaces with the name of one person you love or care for deeply. Rate your agreement with each statement according to the following scale, and enter the appropriate number between 1 and 9.

1	2	3	4	5	6	7	8	9
Not at all				Moderately				Extremely

_____ 1. I am actively supportive of _____'s well-being.

_____ 2. I have a warm relationship with _____.

_____ 3. I am able to count on _____ in times of need.

_____ 4. _____ is able to count on me in times of need.

_____ 5. I am willing to share myself and my possessions with _____.

_____ 6. I receive considerable emotional support from _____.

_____ 7. I give considerable emotional support to _____.

_____ 8. I communicate well with _____.

_____ 9. I value _____ greatly in my life.

_____ 10. I feel close to _____.

_____ 11. I have a comfortable relationship with _____.

_____ 12. I feel that I really understand _____.

_____ 13. I feel that _____ really understands me.

_____ 14. I feel that I can really trust _____.

_____ 15. I share deeply personal information about myself with _____.

_____ 16. Just seeing _____ excites me.

_____ 17. I find myself thinking about _____ frequently during the day.

_____ 18. My relationship with _____ is very romantic.

_____ 19. I find _____ to be very personally attractive.

_____ 20. I idealize _____.

_____ 21. I cannot imagine another person making me as happy as _____ does.

_____ 22. I would rather be with _____ than with anyone else.

_____ 23. There is nothing more important to me than my relationship with _____.

_____ 24. I especially like physical contact with _____.

_____ 25. There is something almost "magical" about my relationship with _____.

_____ 26. I adore _____.

(over)

_____ 27. I cannot imagine life without _____.

_____ 28. My relationship with _____ is passionate.

_____ 29. When I see romantic movies and read romantic books I think of _____.

_____ 30. I fantasize about _____.

_____ 31. I know that I care about _____.

_____ 32. I am committed to maintaining my relationship with _____.

_____ 33. Because of my commitment to _____, I would not let other people come between us.

_____ 34. I have confidence in the stability of my relationship with _____.

_____ 35. I could not let anything get in the way of my commitment to _____.

_____ 36. I expect my love for _____ to last for the rest of my life.

_____ 37. I will always feel a strong responsibility for _____.

_____ 38. I view my commitment to _____ as a solid one.

_____ 39. I cannot imagine ending my relationship with _____.

_____ 40. I am certain of my love for _____.

_____ 41. I view my relationship with _____ as permanent.

_____ 42. I view my relationship with _____ as a good decision.

_____ 43. I feel a sense of responsibility toward _____.

_____ 44. I plan to continue my relationship with _____.

_____ 45. Even when _____ is hard to deal with, I remain committed to our relationship.

Scoring

Psychologist Robert Sternberg sees love as being composed of three components: intimacy, passion, and commitment. The first 15 items in the scale reflect intimacy, the second 15 measure passion, and the final 15 reflect commitment. Add up your scores for each group of 15 items. Find the scores closest to your three totals in the appropriate column below to determine the degree to which you experience each of these three components of love.

Intimacy (Items 1–15)	Passion (Items 16–30)	Commitment (Items 31–45)	
93	73	85	Significantly below average
102	85	96	Somewhat below average
111	98	108	Average
120	110	120	Somewhat above average
129	123	131	Significantly above average

According to Sternberg, high scores in all three components would indicate consummate love. However, uneven or low scores do not necessarily mean that a relationship is not strong: All relationships have ups and downs, and the nature of a relationship may change over time.

WELLNESS WORKSHEET 23

What's Your Gender Communications Quotient?

How much do you know about how men and women communicate with one another? The 20 items in this questionnaire are based on research conducted in classrooms, private homes, businesses, offices, hospitals—the places where people commonly work and socialize. The answers are at the end of this quiz.

	True	False
1. Men talk more than women.	_____	_____
2. Men are more likely to interrupt women than they are to interrupt other men.	_____	_____
3. There are approximately ten times as many sexual terms for males as females in the English language.	_____	_____
4. During conversations, women spend more time gazing at their partner than men do.	_____	_____
5. Nonverbal messages carry more weight than verbal messages.	_____	_____
6. Female managers communicate with more emotional openness and drama than male managers.	_____	_____
7. Men not only control the content of conversations, but they also work harder in keeping conversations going.	_____	_____
8. When people hear generic words such as "mankind" and "he," they respond inclusively, indicating that the terms apply to both sexes.	_____	_____
9. Women are more likely to touch others than men are.	_____	_____
10. In classroom communications, male students receive more reprimands and criticism than female students.	_____	_____
11. Women are more likely than men to disclose information on intimate personal concerns.	_____	_____
12. Female speakers are more animated in their conversational style than are male speakers.	_____	_____
13. Women use less personal space than men.	_____	_____
14. When a male speaks, he is listened to more carefully than a female speaker, even when she makes the identical presentation.	_____	_____
15. In general, women speak in a more tentative style than do men.	_____	_____

(over)

Insel/Roth, *Core Concepts in Health,* Eighth Edition. © 1998 Mayfield Publishing Company. Chapter 4
Insel et al., *Core Concepts in Health,* Brief Eighth Edition. © 1998 Mayfield Publishing Company. Chapter 4

	True	False
16. Women are more likely to answer questions that are not addressed to them.	_____	_____
17. There is widespread sex segregation in schools, and it hinders effective classroom communication.	_____	_____
18. Female managers are seen by both male and female subordinates as better communicators than male managers.	_____	_____
19. In classroom communications, teachers are more likely to give verbal praise to females than to male students.	_____	_____
20. In general, men smile more often than women.	_____	_____

Answers: 1. T; 2. T; 3. F; 4. T; 5. T; 6–9. F; 10–15. T; 16. F; 17. T; 18. T; 19. F; 20. F

SOURCE: Rozema, H. R., Ph.D., and J. W. Gray, Ph.D., Department of Communication, University of Arkansas, Little Rock. Used with permission.

Name _____ Section _____ Date _____

This Family Strengths Inventory was developed by researchers who studied the strengths of over 3000 families. To assess your family (either the family you grew up in or the family you have formed as an adult), circle the number that best reflects how your family rates on each strength. A number 1 represents the lowest rating and a number 5 represents the highest.

1. Spending time together and doing things with each other	1	2	3	4	5
2. Commitment to each other	1	2	3	4	5
3. Good communication (talking with each other often, listening well, sharing feelings with each other)	1	2	3	4	5
4. Dealing with crises in a positive manner	1	2	3	4	5
5. Expressing appreciation to each other	1	2	3	4	5
6. Spiritual wellness	1	2	3	4	5
7. Closeness of relationship between spouses	1	2	3	4	5
8. Closeness of relationship between parents and children	1	2	3	4	5
9. Happiness of relationship between spouses	1	2	3	4	5
10. Happiness of relationship between parents and children	1	2	3	4	5
11. Extent to which spouses make each other feel good about themselves (self-confident, worthy, competent, and happy)	1	2	3	4	5
12. Extent to which parents help children feel good about themselves	1	2	3	4	5

Scoring Add the numbers you have circled. A score below 39 indicates below-average family strengths. Scores between 39 and 52 are in the average range. Scores above 53 indicate a strong family. Low scores on individual items identify areas that families can profitably spend time on. High scores are worthy of celebration but shouldn't lead to complacency. Like gardens, families need loving care to remain strong.

What do you think is your family's major strength? What do you like best about your family?

(over)

Insel/Roth, *Core Concepts in Health,* Eighth Edition. © 1998 Mayfield Publishing Company. Chapter 4
Insel et al., *Core Concepts in Health,* Brief Eighth Edition. © 1998 Mayfield Publishing Company. Chapter 4

What about your family would you most like to change?

WELLNESS WORKSHEET 25

Male and Female Reproductive Systems

Label the parts of the male and female reproductive systems.

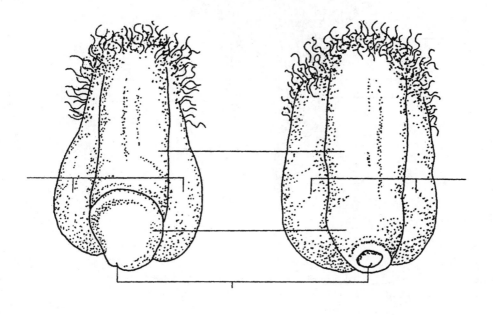

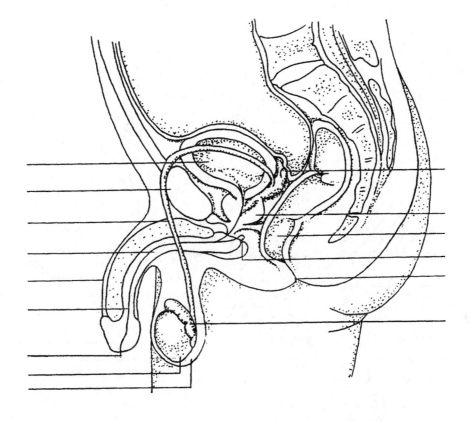

(over)

Insel/Roth, *Core Concepts in Health,* Eighth Edition. © 1998 Mayfield Publishing Company. Chapter 5
Insel et al., *Core Concepts in Health,* Brief Eighth Edition. © 1998 Mayfield Publishing Company. Chapter 5

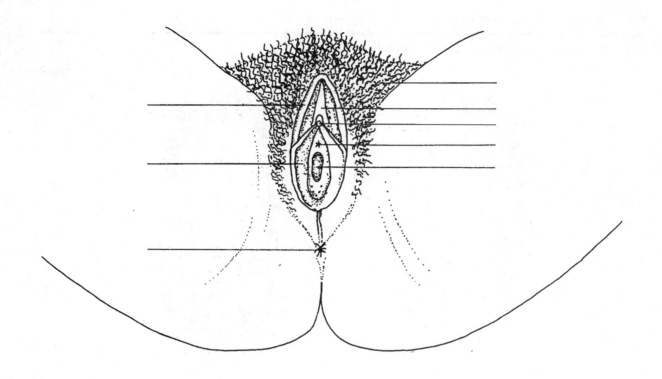

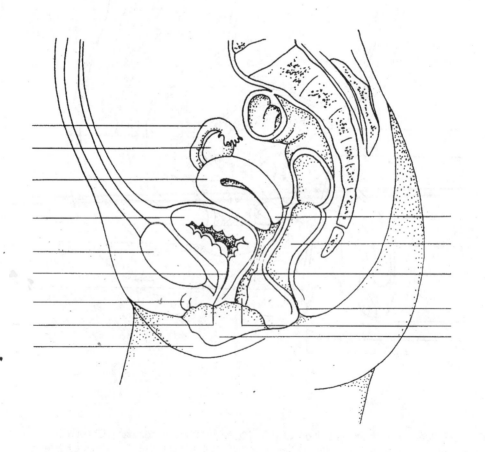

WELLNESS WORKSHEET 26

Test Your Sexual Knowledge and Attitudes

Part I. Your Sexual Knowledge

When 2000 Americans were asked a series of questions about sexuality by the Kinsey Institute, only 45% of the respondents answered more than half the questions correctly. See how you do on this sample of true-or-false questions.

1. The average American first has sexual intercourse at about 16 or 17 years of age. _____

2. About 6 to 8 out of every 10 American women has masturbated. _____

3. Most women have orgasms from penile thrusting alone. _____

4. All men like large female breasts. _____

5. People usually lose interest in sexual activities after age 60. _____

6. Masturbation is physically harmful. _____

7. The average length of a man's erect penis is 5 to 7 inches. _____

8. Impotence usually cannot be treated successfully. _____

9. Petroleum jelly, Vaseline Intensive Care, and baby oil are not good lubricants to use with a diaphragm or condom. _____

10. Most women prefer a sexual partner who has a large penis. _____

11. A woman cannot get pregnant if she has sex during her menstrual period. _____

12. A woman cannot get pregnant if the man withdraws his penis before ejaculating. _____

Answers: 1. T; 2. T; 3. F; 4. F; 5. F; 6. F; 7. T; 8. F; 9. T; 10. F; 11. F; 12. F

How well did you score? If you're not satisfied with your level of knowledge, consider checking your local library or bookstore for reputable self-help books about sexual functioning.

(over)

Insel/Roth, *Core Concepts in Health*, Eighth Edition. © 1998 Mayfield Publishing Company. Chapter 5
Insel et al., *Core Concepts in Health*, Brief Eighth Edition. © 1998 Mayfield Publishing Company. Chapter 5

Part II. Your Sexual Attitudes

For each statement, circle the response that most closely reflects your position.

	Agree	Not sure	Disagree
1. Sex education encourages young people to have sex.	1	2	3
2. Homosexuality is a healthy, normal expression of sexuality.	3	2	1
3. Members of the other sex will think more highly of you if you remain mysterious.	1	2	3
4. It's better to wait until marriage to have sex.	1	2	3
5. Abortion should be a personal, private choice for a woman.	3	2	1
6. It's natural for men to have more sexual freedom than women.	1	2	3
7. Condoms should not be made available to teenagers.	1	2	3
8. Pornography should not be restricted for adults.	3	2	1
9. A woman who is raped usually does something to provoke it.	1	2	3
10. Contraception is the woman's responsibility.	1	2	3
11. Feminism has had a positive influence on society.	3	2	1
12. Masturbation is a healthy expression of sexuality.	3	2	1
13. I have many friends of the other sex.	3	2	1
14. Prostitution should be legalized.	3	2	1
15. Women use sex for love, men use love for sex.	1	2	3
16. Our society is too sexually permissive.	1	2	3
17. The man should be the undisputed head of the household.	1	2	3
18. Having sex just for pleasure is OK.	3	2	1

Scoring

Add up the numbers you circled to obtain your overall score. Find your score and rating below.

1–18	Traditional attitude about sexuality
19–36	Ambivalent or mixed attitude about sexuality
37–54	Open, progressive attitude about sexuality

PART I QUIZ SOURCE: Adapted from Reinisch, J. M., and R. Beasley. 1990. *The Kinsey Institute New Report on Sex.* (New York: St. Martin's Press. Copyright © 1990 St Martin's Press, Inc.

WELLNESS WORKSHEET 27

Gender Roles

In the spaces provided below, list ten characteristics and behaviors that you associate with being male and female in our society.

Male	**Female**
1. _____	1. _____
2. _____	2. _____
3. _____	3. _____
4. _____	4. _____
5. _____	5. _____
6. _____	6. _____
7. _____	7. _____
8. _____	8. _____
9. _____	9. _____
10. _____	10. _____

Circle the numbers of ten characteristics from the twenty that you feel best apply to yourself.
Did you choose any characteristics from your list for the other sex? If so, how many? _____

If you found most of the characteristics you chose for yourself were from your list for your own sex, are there any characteristics from the other list you wish you did have? Do you feel our society's definitions of gender roles are preventing you from behaving or developing in the ways you'd most like to?

(over)

Insel/Roth, *Core Concepts in Health*, Eighth Edition. © 1998 Mayfield Publishing Company. Chapter 5
Insel et al., *Core Concepts in Health*, Brief Eighth Edition. © 1998 Mayfield Publishing Company. Chapter 4

If the characteristics you chose for yourself were a mix of both lists, what do you think your description of yourself indicates about the prevailing ideas about male and female characteristics you described for our society? How valid are they?

Name _____ Section _____ Date _____

Facts About Contraception

To help you choose the best method of contraception for you and your partner, you must first be familiar with the different methods. Fill in the boxes below with the advantages and disadvantages of each method, along with how well each one protects against pregnanacy and STDs. Use your text if necessary.

Method	Advantages	Disadvantages	Effectiveness/ STD protection
Oral contraceptives			
Norplant implants			
Depo-Provera injections			
IUD			
Male condom			
Female condom			

(over)

Insel/Roth, *Core Concepts in Health*, Eighth Edition. © 1998 Mayfield Publishing Company. Chapter 6
Insel et al., *Core Concepts in Health*, Brief Eighth Edition. © 1998 Mayfield Publishing Company. Chapter 6

Method	Advantages	Disadvantages	Effectiveness/ STD protection
Diaphragm with spermicide			
Cervical cap			
Vaginal spermicides			
FAM			
Male sterilization			
Female sterilization			

Name _____ Section _____ Date _____

WELLNESS WORKSHEET 29

Which Contraceptive Method Is Right for You and Your Partner?

If you are sexually active, you need to use the contraceptive method that will work best for you. A number of factors may be involved in your decision. The following questions will help you sort out these factors and choose an appropriate method. Answer yes (Y) or no (N) for each statement as it applies to you and, if appropriate, your partner.

Y or N

_____ 1. I like sexual spontaneity and don't want to be bothered with contraception at the time of sexual intercourse.

_____ 2. I need a contraceptive immediately.

_____ 3. It is very important that I do not become pregnant now.

_____ 4. I want a contraceptive method that will protect me and my partner against STDs.

_____ 5. I prefer a contraceptive method that requires the cooperation and involvement of both partners.

_____ 6. I have sexual intercourse frequently.

_____ 7. I have sexual intercourse infrequently.

_____ 8. I am forgetful or have a variable daily routine.

_____ 9. I have more than one sexual partner.

_____ 10. I have heavy periods with cramps.

_____ 11. I prefer a method that requires little or no action or bother on my part.

_____ 12. I am a nursing mother.

_____ 13. I want the option of conceiving immediately after discontinuing contraception.

_____ 14. I want a contraceptive method with few or no side effects.

If you answered "yes" to the numbers of statements listed on the left, the method on the right might be a good choice for you:

1, 3, 6, 10, 11	Oral contraceptives
1, 3, 6, 8, 10, 11	Norplant
1, 3, 6, 8, 10, 11, 12	Depo-Provera
1, 3, 6, 8, 11, 12, 13	IUD
2, 4, 5, 7, 8, 9, 12, 13, 14	Condoms (male and female)
5, 7, 12, 13, 14	Diaphragm and spermicide
5, 7, 12, 13, 14	Cervical cap
2, 5, 7, 8, 12, 13, 14	Vaginal spermicides
5, 7, 13, 14	FAM

Your answers may indicate that more than one method would be appropriate for you. To help narrow your choices, circle the numbers of the statements that are *most* important for you. Before you make a final choice, talk with your partner(s) and your physician. Consider your own lifestyle and preferences as well as characteristics of each method (effectiveness, side effects, costs, and so on). For maximum protection against pregnancy and STDs, you might want to consider combining two methods.

(over)

Insel/Roth, *Core Concepts in Health,* Eighth Edition. © 1998 Mayfield Publishing Company. Chapter 6
Insel et al., *Core Concepts in Health,* Brief Eighth Edition. © 1998 Mayfield Publishing Company. Chapter 6

INTERNET ACTIVITY

To help in your decision about contraception, research one of the methods that the quiz indicated would be appropriate for you and your partner. Visit one of the following sites, or do a search. (If you want further guidance in choosing a method, take the interactive contraception questionnaire located at the Web site for the Association of Reproductive Health Professionals: http://www.arhp.org/)

Planned Parenthood Federation of America: http://www.ppfa.org/ppfa

Ann Rose's Ultimate Birth Control Links Page: http://gynpages.com/ultimate

Office of Population Affairs: http://www.dhhs.gov/progorg/opa

Contraceptive method to investigate:_____

Site visited (URL):_____

What new information about the method did you find?

Has what you've learned made you more or less likely to choose this method? Why?

What other useful information or materials does the site provide?

WELLNESS WORKSHEET 30

Facts About Methods of Abortion

Familiarize yourself with the different methods of abortion by completing the chart below. Refer to your text-book if necessary.

Method	Description of procedure	Potential side effects	Time in pregnancy when used
Vacuum aspiration			
Menstrual extraction			
Dilation and evacuation			
RU-486			

(over)

Insel/Roth, *Core Concepts in Health,* Eighth Edition. © 1998 Mayfield Publishing Company. Chapter 7

Method	Description of procedure	Potential side effects	Time in pregnancy when used
Saline instillation			
Prostaglandins			

✍ WELLNESS WORKSHEET 31

Your Position on the Legality and Morality of Abortion

To help define your own position on abortion, answer the following series of questions.

	Agree	Disagree
1. The fertilized egg is a human being from the moment of conception.	_____	_____
2. The rights of the fetus at any stage take precedence over any decision a woman might want to make regarding her pregnancy.	_____	_____
3. The rights of the fetus depend upon its gestational age: further along in the pregnancy, the fetus has more rights.	_____	_____
4. Each individual woman should have final say over decisions regarding her health and body; politicians should not be allowed to decide.	_____	_____
5. In cases of teenagers seeking an abortion, parental consent should be required.	_____	_____
6. In cases of married women seeking an abortion, spousal consent should be required.	_____	_____
7. In cases of late abortion, tests should be done to determine the viability of the fetus.	_____	_____
8. The federal government should provide public funding for abortion to ensure equal access to abortion for all women.	_____	_____
9. The federal government should not allow states to pass their own abortion laws; there should be uniform laws for the entire country.	_____	_____

10. Does a woman's right to choose whether or not to have an abortion depend upon the circumstances surrounding conception or the situation of the mother? In which of the following situations, if any, would you support a woman's right to choose to have an abortion (check where appropriate):

_____ An abortion is necessary to maintain the woman's life or health.

_____ The pregnancy is a result of rape or incest.

_____ A serious birth defect has been detected in the fetus.

_____ The pregnancy is a result of the failure of a contraceptive method or device.

_____ The pregnancy occurred when no contraceptive method was in use.

_____ A single mother, pregnant for the fifth time, wants an abortion because she feels she cannot support another child.

_____ A pregnant 15-year-old high school student feels having a child would be too great a disruption in her life and keep her from reaching her goals for the future.

_____ A pregnant 19-year-old college student does not want to interrupt her education.

_____ The father of the child has stated he will provide no support and is not interested in helping raise the child.

_____ Parents of two boys wish to terminate the mother's pregnancy because the fetus is male rather than female.

(over)

On the basis of your answers to the questions on the previous page, write out your position on abortion. Should it be legal or illegal? Are there certain circumstances in which it should or should not be allowed? What sorts of rules should govern when it can be performed?

INTERNET ACTIVITY

To further develop your own position on abortion, review the materials at Web sites sponsored by a pro-life and a pro-choice group; use the sites listed in your text or do a search. Explore each site and note down here any arguments or points that you haven't previously considered.

URL of pro-life group sponsored site:_____
New arguments:

URL of pro-choice group sponsored site:_____
New arguments:

Name _____ Section _____ Date _____

WELLNESS WORKSHEET 32

Assessing Your Readiness to Become a Parent

Many factors have to be taken into account when you are considering parenthood. The following are some questions you should ask yourself and some issues you should consider when making this decision. Some issues are relevant to both men and women; others apply only to women. There are no "right" answers—you must decide for yourself what your answers reveal about your aptitude for parenthood.

Yes   No

Physical Health

____ ____ 1. Are you in reasonably good health?

____ ____ 2. Do you have any behaviors or conditions that could be of special concern?

____ Obesity	____ Anemia
____ Smoking	____ Diabetes
____ Alcohol and drug use	____ Sexually transmitted diseases
____ Hypertension	____ Epilepsy
____ Previous problems with pregnancy or delivery	____ Prenatal exposure to diethylstilbestrol (DES)
	____ Asthma

____ ____ 3. Are you under 20 or over 35 years of age?

____ ____ 4. Do you or your partner have a family history of a genetic problem that a baby might inherit?

____ Hemophilia	____ Phenylketonuria (PKU)
____ Sickle cell disease	____ Cystic fibrosis
____ Down syndrome	____ Thalassemia
____ Tay-Sachs disease	____ Other

Financial Circumstances

____ ____ 1. Will your health insurance cover the costs of pregnancy, prenatal tests, delivery, and medical attention for the mother and baby before and after the birth?

____ ____ 2. Can you afford the supplies for the baby: diapers, bedding, crib, stroller, car seat, clothing, food, and medical supplies?

____ ____ 3. Will one parent leave his or her job to care for the baby?

____ ____ 4. If so, can the decrease in family income be worked into the family budget?

____ ____ 5. If both parents will continue to work, has affordable child care been set up?

____ ____ 6. The annual cost of raising a child is about $7500; can you save and/or provide the necessary money?

Education, Career, and Child Care Plans

____ ____ 1. Have you completed as much of your education as you want?

____ ____ 2. Have you sufficiently established yourself in a career, if that is important to you?

____ ____ 3. Have you investigated parental leave and company-sponsored child care?

____ ____ 4. Do both spouses agree on child care arrangements?

(over)

Insel/Roth, *Core Concepts in Health,* Eighth Edition. © 1998 Mayfield Publishing Company. Chapter 8
Insel et al., *Core Concepts in Health,* Brief Eighth Edition. © 1998 Mayfield Publishing Company. Chapter 4

Yes **No**

Lifestyle and Social Support

____ ____ 1. Would you be willing to give up the freedom to do what you want to do when you want to do it?

____ ____ 2. Would you be willing to restrict your social life, to lose leisure time and privacy?

____ ____ 3. Would you and your partner be prepared to spend more time at home? Would you have enough time to spend with a child?

____ ____ 4. Are you prepared to be a single parent if your partner leaves or dies?

____ ____ 5. Do you have a network of family and friends who will help you with the baby? Are there community resources you can call on for additional assistance?

Readiness

____ ____ 1. Are you prepared to have a helpless being completely dependent on you 24 hours a day?

____ ____ 2. Do you like children? Have you enough experiences with babies, toddlers, and teenagers?

____ ____ 3. Do you think time spent with children is time well spent?

____ ____ 4. Do you communicate easily with others?

____ ____ 5. Do you have enough love to give a child? Can you express affection easily?

____ ____ 6. Do you feel good enough about yourself to respect and nurture others?

____ ____ 7. Do you have safe ways of handling anger, frustration, and impatience?

____ ____ 8. Would you be willing to devote a great part of your life, at least 18 years, to being responsible for a child?

Relationship with Partner

____ ____ 1. Does your partner want to have a child? Is he or she willing to ask these same questions of himself or herself?

____ ____ 2. Have you adequately discussed your reasons for wanting a child?

____ ____ 3. Does either of you have philosophical objections to adding to the world's population?

____ ____ 4. Have you and your partner discussed each other's feelings about religion, work, family, and child raising? Are your feelings compatible and conducive to good parenting?

____ ____ 5. Would both you and your partner contribute in raising the child?

____ ____ 6. Is your relationship stable? Could you provide a child with a really good home environment?

____ ____ 7. After having a child, would your partner and you be able to separate if you should have unsolvable problems? Would you feel obligated to remain together for the sake of the child?

WELLNESS WORKSHEET 33

Facts About Pregnancy and Childbirth

Review your knowledge of pregnancy and childbirth by answering the questions below. Refer to your textbook if necessary.

Conception

1. Trace the journey of the egg in a woman's body:

    _____   ovary   ⟶   _____   ⟶   _____   ⟶   _____ (fertilized)

    ↘ _____ (unfertilized)

    How long does the egg's journey take? _____

2. Trace the journey of sperm cells from ejaculation to conception:

    _____   penis   ⟶   _____   ⟶   _____   ⟶   _____   ⟶   _____

    How does a sperm cell penetrate an egg? _____

    _____

3. List three possible reasons for infertility in women.

    a. _____

    b. _____

    c. _____

    List two possible reasons for infertility in men.

    a. _____

    b. _____

4. List and define four treatments for infertility.

    a. _____

    b. _____

    c. _____

    d. _____

Pregnancy

1. List three early signs and symptoms of pregnancy.

    a. _____

    b. _____

    c. _____

(over)

Insel/Roth, *Core Concepts in Health,* Eighth Edition. © 1998 Mayfield Publishing Company. Chapter 8
Insel et al., *Core Concepts in Health,* Brief Eighth Edition. © 1998 Mayfield Publishing Company. Chapter 5

2. List specific changes that occur in the following during pregnancy.

uterus _____

breasts _____

muscles and ligaments _____

pelvic joints _____

circulatory system _____

kidneys _____

body weight _____

emotions _____

3. What are Braxton Hicks contractions? When do they occur and why?

_____

_____

4. List three characteristics of the fetus during each trimester. What systems have developed? How large is the fetus?

first trimester	second trimester	third trimester
_____	_____	_____
_____	_____	_____
_____	_____	_____

5. List six important components of good prenatal care.

a. _____   d. _____

b. _____   e. _____

c. _____   f. _____

Childbirth

What occurs during each of the three stages of labor? How long does each stage last?

first stage: _____

second stage: _____

third stage: _____

Name _____ Section _____ Date _____

WELLNESS WORKSHEET 34

Creating a Family Health Tree

Knowing that a specific disease runs in your family allows you to watch closely for the early warning signs and get appropriate screening tests. It can also help you target important health habits to adopt. You can put together a simple family health tree by compiling key facts on your primary relatives: siblings, parents, aunts and uncles, and grandparents. If possible, have your primary relatives fill out a family health history record like the one below.

Family Health History

Name _____   Date of birth _____

Blood and Rh type: _____   Occupation: _____

Please note any serious or chronic diseases you have experienced, with special attention to the following:

_____ Alcoholism

_____ Allergies

_____ Arthritis

_____ Asthma

_____ Blood diseases (hemophilia, sickle cell disease, thalassemia)

_____ Cancer (breast, bowel, colon, ovarian, skin, stomach, etc.)

_____ Cystic fibrosis

_____ Diabetes

_____ Epilepsy

_____ Familial high blood cholesterol levels

_____ Hearing defects

_____ Heart defects

_____ Huntington's disease

_____ Hypertension (high blood pressure)

_____ Learning disabilities (dyslexia, attention deficit disorder, autism)

_____ Liver disease (particularly hepatitis)

_____ Lupus

_____ Mental illness (manic depressive disorders, schizophrenia)

_____ Mental impairment (Down syndrome, fragile X, etc.)

_____ Migraine headaches

_____ Miscarriages or neonatal deaths

_____ Multiple sclerosis

_____ Muscular dystrophy

_____ Myasthenia gravis

_____ Obesity

_____ Phenylketonuria (PKU)

_____ Respiratory disease (emphysema, bacterial pneumonia)

_____ Rh disease

_____ Skin disorders (particularly psoriasis)

_____ Thyroid disorders

_____ Tay-Sachs disease

_____ Tuberculosis

_____ Visual disorders (dyslexia, glaucoma, retinitis pigmentosa)

_____ Other (please list):

(over)

Insel/Roth, *Core Concepts in Health,* Eighth Edition. © 1998 Mayfield Publishing Company. Chapter 8
Insel et al., *Core Concepts in Health,* Brief Eighth Edition. © 1998 Mayfield Publishing Company. Chapter 5

List any important health-related behaviors (including tobacco use, dietary and exercise habits, and alcohol use):

Please note names of your relatives below, along with indications of any illnesses, such as those listed on the previous page, which affected them. If deceased, list age and cause. Also make note of lifestyle habits such as smoking.

Father: _____

_____

Mother: _____

_____

Brothers and sisters: _____

_____

Children of brothers and sisters: _____

_____

_____

If you don't have enough information on past generations, you can get clues by requesting death certificates from state health departments or medical records from relatives' physicians or hospitals where they died. Once you've collected the information you want, plug it into the tree format as shown in your text.

WELLNESS WORKSHEET 35

Developing a Birth Plan

What type of birth experience would you and your partner prefer? Think about your preferences in each of the following areas. In addition to considering these questions on your own and with your partner, you would also need to discuss them with your physician or midwife.

1. Who will be present at the birth? The father? Friends? Children or other relatives?

2. What type of room would you like to be in for the birth?

3. What type of environment—music, lighting, furniture, and so on—would you prefer?

4. Who would you like to have "catch" the baby when he or she is born? Who will cut the umbilical cord?

5. Will the baby be fed by breast or bottle?

(over)

Insel/Roth, *Core Concepts in Health,* Eighth Edition. © 1998 Mayfield Publishing Company. Chapter 8
Insel et al., *Core Concepts in Health,* Brief Eighth Edition. © 1998 Mayfield Publishing Company. Chapter 5

6. What types of routine medical tests and treatments may be performed? (These are questions that should be discussed with your physician or midwife.)

- Can the mother eat or drink during labor?

- Can the mother take a shower or bath during labor? Walk around?

- Under what circumstances would drugs be used to induce or augment labor?

- Is electronic fetal monitoring used?

- Under what circumstances would an episiotomy be performed?

- Under what circumstances would forceps or vacuum extraction be used?

- What types of medications are typically used during labor and delivery?

- Under what circumstances would a cesarean section be performed?

- Can the baby spend the night in the mother's room rather than in the nursery?

Name _____ Section _____ Date _____

Part I. General Addictive Behavior Checklist

Choose an activity or behavior in your life that you feel may be developing into an addiction. Ask yourself the following questions about it, and answer yes (Y) or no (N).

Activity/behavior: _____

_____ 1. Do you engage in the activity on a regular basis?

_____ 2. Have you engaged in the activity over a long period of time?

_____ 3. Do you currently engage in this activity more than you used to?

_____ 4. Do you find it difficult to stop or to avoid the activity?

_____ 5. Have you tried and failed to cut down on the amount of time you spend on the activity?

_____ 6. Do you turn down or skip social/recreational events in order to engage in the activity?

_____ 7. Does your participation in the activity interfere with your attendance and/or performance at school and/or work?

_____ 8. Have friends or family members spoken to you about the activity and indicated they think you have a problem?

_____ 9. Has your participation in the activity affected your reputation?

_____ 10. Have you lied to friends or family members about the amount of time, money, and other resources that you put into the activity?

_____ 11. Do you feel guilty about the resources that you put into the activity?

_____ 12. Do you engage in the activity when you are worried, frustrated, or stressed or when you have other painful feelings?

_____ 13. Do you feel better when you engage in the activity?

_____ 14. Do you often spend more time engaged in the activity than you plan to?

_____ 15. Do you have a strong urge to participate in the activity when you are away from it?

_____ 16. Do you spend a lot of time planning for your next opportunities to engage in the activity?

_____ 17. Are you often irritable and restless when you are away from the activity?

_____ 18. Do you use the activity as a reward for all other accomplishments?

(over)

Insel/Roth, *Core Concepts in Health*, Eighth Edition. © 1998 Mayfield Publishing Company. Chapter 9
Insel et al., *Core Concepts in Health*, Brief Eighth Edition. © 1998 Mayfield Publishing Company. Chapter 7

Part II. Checklist for Drug Dependency

If you wonder whether you are becoming dependent on a drug, ask yourself the following questions. Answer yes (Y) or no (N).

_____ 1. Do you take the drug on a regular basis?

_____ 2. Have you been taking the drug for a long time?

_____ 3. Do you always take the drug in certain situations or when you're with certain people?

_____ 4. Do you find it difficult to stop using the drug? Do you feel powerless to quit?

_____ 5. Have you tried repeatedly to cut down or control your use of the drug?

_____ 6. Do you need to take a larger dose of the drug in order to get the same high you're used to?

_____ 7. Do you feel specific symptoms if you cut back or stop using the drug?

_____ 8. Do you frequently take another psychoactive substance to relieve withdrawal symptoms?

_____ 9. Do you take the drug to feel "normal"?

_____ 10. Do you go to extreme lengths or put yourself in dangerous situations to get the drug?

_____ 11. Do you hide your drug use from others? Have you ever lied about what you're using or how much you use?

_____ 12. Do people close to you ask you about your drug use?

_____ 13. Are you spending more and more time with people who use the drug you use?

_____ 14. Do you think about the drug when you're not high, figuring out ways to get it?

_____ 15. If you stop taking the drug, do you feel bad until you can take it again?

_____ 16. Does the drug interfere with your ability to study, work, or socialize?

_____ 17. Do you skip important school, occupational, social, or recreational activities in order to obtain or use the drug?

_____ 18. Do you continue to use the drug despite a physical or mental disorder or despite a significant problem that you know is worsened by drug use?

_____ 19. Have you developed a mental or physical condition or disorder because of prolonged drug use?

_____ 20. Have you done something dangerous or that you regret while under the influence of the drug?

Evaluation

On each of these checklists, the more times you answer yes, the more likely it is that you are developing an addiction. If your answers suggest abuse or dependency, talk to someone at your school health clinic or to your physician about taking care of the problem before it gets worse.

Name _____ Section _____ Date _____

WELLNESS WORKSHEET 37

Reasons for Using or Not Using Drugs

If you have tried a psychoactive drug in the past, describe the circumstances of your first use of the drug. What were your reasons for trying the drug? Did other people have an effect on your decision to try the drug? Did you seek out the experience, or did you find yourself in a situation where the drug was available?

If you have continued to use a psychoactive drug, what are your reasons? Which of the following apply to you?

_____ 1. Taking drugs allows me to escape boredom or depression.

_____ 2. Drug use allows me to socialize with a group of people with whom I want to socialize.

_____ 3. Using drugs makes me feel daring.

_____ 4. Using drugs is exciting because they are illicit.

_____ 5. Drug use makes me feel better about myself.

_____ 6. Taking drugs allows me to alter my mood or see the world in a way I can't without the drugs.

_____ 7. Drug use is a natural part of my society.

_____ 8. I take drugs to rebel against my parents or society.

_____ 9. Drug use is enjoyable.

_____ 10. Drugs allow me to socialize more easily.

_____ 11. Drug use allows me to be a more spiritual person.

_____ 12. I take drugs when I am angry or upset.

List other reasons that apply to you.

(over)

Insel/Roth, *Core Concepts in Health,* Eighth Edition. © 1998 Mayfield Publishing Company. Chapter 9
Insel et al., *Core Concepts in Health,* Brief Eighth Edition. © 1998 Mayfield Publishing Company. Chapter 7

If you have never tried a psychoactive drug, give your reasons for this choice.

If you have been in a situation where you were offered a psychoactive drug and turned it down, what reasons did you give? What would you say to someone who asked you why you were refusing the drug? Can you offer suggestions to someone who does not want to use psychoactive drugs but feels self-conscious about refusing them when they are offered?

INTERNET ACTIVITY

Use the Internet to find out more about a psychoactive drug that you've tried or been offered. Try one or more of the sites listed below or use a search engine to find other useful sites.

Web of Addictions: http://www.well.com/user/woa

National Clearinghouse for Alcohol and Drug Information: http://www.health.org/

Healthtouch: http://www.healthtouch.com/level1/leaflets/102504/102504.htm

Drug researched:_____

Site(s) visited (URL):_____

What new information did you find about the short- and long-term effects of the drug?

Write a brief description of the most helpful or interesting site you visited. What information and resources does the site provide?

Name _____ Section _____ Date _____

WELLNESS WORKSHEET 38

Facts About Psychoactive Drugs

Familiarize yourself with the different types of psychoactive drugs by filling in the blanks below; refer to your textbook as needed.

Opioids

Major drugs: _____

Routes of intake: _____

_____

Effects: _____

_____

_____

Special problems associated with use (overdose, tolerance, withdrawal, injuries, crime): _____

_____

Central Nervous System Depressants

Major drugs: _____

Routes of intake: _____

_____

Effects: _____

_____

_____

Special problems associated with use (overdose, tolerance, withdrawal, injuries, crime): _____

_____

Central Nervous System Stimulants

Major drugs: _____

Routes of intake: _____

_____

Effects: _____

_____

_____

Special problems associated with use (overdose, tolerance, withdrawal, injuries, crime): _____

_____

_____

Marijuana and Other Cannabis Products

Major drugs: _____

Routes of intake: _____

_____

Effects: _____

_____

_____

Special problems associated with use (overdose, tolerance, withdrawal, injuries, crime): _____

_____

_____

Hallucinogens

Major drugs: _____

Routes of intake: _____

_____

_____

Effects: _____

_____

Special problems associated with use (overdose, tolerance, withdrawal, injuries, crime): _____

_____

_____

Inhalants

Major drugs: _____

Routes of intake: _____

_____

Effects: _____

_____

_____

Special problems associated with use (overdose, tolerance, withdrawal, injuries, crime): _____

_____

_____

WELLNESS WORKSHEET 39

Is Alcohol a Problem in Your Life?

Part I. Do You Have a Problem with Alcohol?

To determine if you or someone close to you may have a drinking problem, complete the CAGE screening test by answering yes or no to the following questions:

Have you ever felt you should . . . . . Cut down on your drinking?

Have people . . . . Annoyed you by criticizing your drinking?

Have you ever felt bad or . . . . Guilty about your drinking?

Have you ever had an . . . . Eye-opener (a drink first thing in the morning to steady
your nerves or get rid of a hangover)?

One "yes" response suggests a possible alcohol problem. If you answered yes to more than one question, it is highly likely that a problem exists. In either case, it is important that you see your physician or other health care provider right away to discuss your responses to these questions. Even if you answered no to all of the above questions, if you are encountering drinking-related problems with your job, academic performance, relationships, or health, or with the law, you should still seek professional help.

Part II. Are You Troubled by Someone Else's Drinking?

Millions of people are affected by the excessive drinking of someone close to them. The following checklist was created by Al-Anon to help people determine whether they are adversely affected by someone else's drinking. Check any statement that is true for you.

_____ 1. Do you worry about how much someone drinks?

_____ 2. Do you have money problems because of someone else's drinking?

_____ 3. Do you tell lies to cover up for someone else's drinking?

_____ 4. Do you feel that if the drinker loved you, he or she would stop drinking to please you?

_____ 5. Do you blame the drinker's behavior on his or her companions?

_____ 6. Are plans frequently upset or canceled or meals delayed because of the drinker?

_____ 7. Do you make threats, such as, "If you don't stop drinking, I'll leave you"?

_____ 8. Do you secretly try to smell the drinker's breath?

_____ 9. Are you afraid to upset someone for fear it will set off a drinking bout?

_____ 10. Have you been hurt or embarrassed by the drinker's behavior?

_____ 11. Are holidays and gatherings spoiled because of drinking?

_____ 12. Have you considered calling the police for help in fear of abuse?

_____ 13. Do you search for hidden alcohol?

(over)

Insel/Roth, *Core Concepts in Health,* Eighth Edition. © 1998 Mayfield Publishing Company. Chapter 10
Insel et al., *Core Concepts in Health,* Brief Eighth Edition. © 1998 Mayfield Publishing Company. Chapter 8

_____ 14. Do you often ride in a car with a driver who has been drinking?

_____ 15. Have you refused social invitations out of fear or anxiety?

_____ 16. Do you sometimes feel like a failure when you think of the lengths you have gone to control the drinker?

_____ 17. Do you think that if the drinker stopped drinking, your other problems would be solved?

_____ 18. Do you ever threaten to hurt yourself to scare the drinker?

_____ 19. Do you feel angry, confused, or depressed most of the time?

_____ 20. Do you feel there is no one who understands your problems?

If your responses indicate that you are affected by the drinking of someone close to you, consider contacting Al-Anon for help:

Al-Anon Family Group Headquarters, Inc.
1600 Corporate Landing Parkway
Virginia Beach, VA 23454-5617
800-344-2666
http://www.al-anon.alateen.org

SOURCES: CAGE test: National Institute on Alcohol Abuse and Alcoholism. 1996. *Alcoholism: Getting the Facts.* NIH Publication No. 96–4153. Drinking checklist: Are You Troubled By Someone's Drinking? (http://www.al-anon.alateen.org/quiz.html) Copyright © 1980 Al-Anon Family Group Headquarters, Inc. Reprinted by permission of Al-Anon Family Group Headquarters, Inc.

WELLNESS WORKSHEET 40

Alcohol and How It Affects You

Evaluate Your Reasons for Drinking

Be honest with yourself. It is necessary for you to know why you drink in order to control your alcohol-related behavior. Put a check next to the statements that are true for you.

I drink to tune myself in to

_____ enhance enjoyment of people, activities, special occasions

_____ promote social ease by relaxing inhibitions, aiding ability to talk and relate to others

_____ complement and add to enjoyment of food

_____ relax after a period of hard work and/or tension

I drink to tune myself out to

_____ escape problems

_____ mask fears when courage and self-confidence are lacking

_____ block out painful loneliness, self-doubt, feelings of inadequacy

_____ substitute for close relationships, challenging activity

_____ mask a sense of guilt about drinking

Alcohol Content

Drinks differ in the amount of pure alcohol they contain; therefore, a "drink" means different amounts of liquid depending on the type of drink. A proof value indicates concentration of alcohol in a particular drink; the proof value is equal to twice the percentage of alcohol in a drink. To calculate the number of ounces of pure alcohol in a drink, multiply the size of the drink by the percentage of alcohol it contains (one-half proof value). For example, a 12 oz. beer (10 proof) has 0.6 oz. of pure alcohol (10 proof = 5% alcohol concentration; 0.05×12 oz. = 0.6 oz.).

Calculate the number of ounces of pure alcohol in each of the following drinks.

Drink	Size (oz.)	Proof value	Ounces of pure alcohol
beer	12	10	_____
wine	6	24	_____
sherry	4	40	_____
liquor	1.5	80	_____

Try the calculations on different size drinks and drinks of different alcohol content.

_____	_____	_____	_____
_____	_____	_____	_____
_____	_____	_____	_____
_____	_____	_____	_____

(over)

Insel/Roth, *Core Concepts in Health*, Eighth Edition. © 1998 Mayfield Publishing Company. Chapter 10
Insel et al., *Core Concepts in Health*, Brief Eighth Edition. © 1998 Mayfield Publishing Company. Chapter 8

Maintenance Rate (or how long to sip a drink)

Remember that the effects of alcohol will be greater when your BAC is rising than when you keep it stable or allow it to fall. BAC is directly proportional to the rate of ethyl alcohol intake. Assuming a general maintenance rate (rate at which the body rids itself of alcohol) of 0.1 oz. of pure alcohol per hour per 50 pounds of body weight, you can calculate the approximate length of time it takes you to metabolize a given drink by applying the following formula:

$$\frac{2.5 \times \text{proof of drink} \times \text{volume (size in oz.) of drink}}{\text{body weight}} = \text{time in hours per drink}$$

For example, to calculate how long it will take to metabolize one can (12 oz.) of 10-proof beer for a person weighing 150 pounds:

$$\frac{2.5 \times 10 \times 12}{150} = 2 \text{ hours}$$

So, it takes this 150-pound individual 2 hours to completely metabolize one 12 oz. can of 10-proof beer.

Choose your favorite three drinks (or choose three of the examples from the previous page) and use this formula to calculate your maintenance rate for each drink.

1. $\dfrac{(\quad) \times (\quad) \times (\quad)}{(\quad)} =$ ┌─────────────────┐ │ hours/drink │ └─────────────────┘

2. $\dfrac{(\quad) \times (\quad) \times (\quad)}{(\quad)} =$ ┌─────────────────┐ │ hours/drink │ └─────────────────┘

3. $\dfrac{(\quad) \times (\quad) \times (\quad)}{(\quad)} =$ ┌─────────────────┐ │ hours/drink │ └─────────────────┘

In Case of Excess

To sober up, the only remedy that works is to stop drinking and allow time. For any given type of drink, the amount of time would be the number of drinks you have consumed multiplied by your maintenance rate for that drink. For the example given above, if the 150-pound individual had consumed three 12 oz. cans of 10-proof beer, he or she would have to wait 6 hours before the alcohol would be metabolized. Calculate the amount of time that would have to elapse for you to metabolize all the alcohol if you had consumed three of one of the types of drinks you calculated a maintenance rate for above:

$$3 \times (\quad\quad) = \underline{\quad\quad\quad} \text{ hours}$$

Given this consumption level, your answer here indicates the number of hours you should wait before driving.

WELLNESS WORKSHEET 41

Drinking and Driving

Protecting Yourself on the Road

List eight signs of an impaired driver.

1._____   5._____

2._____   6._____

3._____   7._____

4._____   8._____

List strategies for the following situations in which you encounter an impaired driver.

1. The driver is ahead of you.

2. The driver is behind you.

3. The driver is approaching you.

Being a Responsible Guest

List four strategies for drinking less in a social situation or for avoiding driving while impaired.

1._____

2._____

3._____

4._____

Create a schedule or plan below for sharing designated driver responsibilities.

_____

_____

_____

_____

(over)

Insel/Roth, *Core Concepts in Health,* Eighth Edition. © 1998 Mayfield Publishing Company. Chapter 10
Insel et al., *Core Concepts in Health,* Brief Eighth Edition. © 1998 Mayfield Publishing Company. Chapter 8

Being a Responsible Host

List four strategies for seeing that your guests do not leave your home or residence while impaired.

1._____

2._____

3._____

4._____

List three things you might say or do for someone who is leaving your residence impaired and insists on driving home.

1._____

2._____

3._____

INTERNET ACTIVITY

Research additional strategies for preventing drunk driving—for drinking moderately, if at all, in social situations; for using designated drivers; and/or for being a responsible party host. Visit the sites listed below or use a search engine to locate other useful sites.

Higher Education Center for Alcohol and Other Drug Prevention: http://www.edc.org/hec
Habitsmart: http://www.cts.com/crash/habtsmrt/
Indiana University Alcohol and Drug Information Center: http://www.indiana.edu/~adic/
Go Ask Alice: http://www.columbia.edu/cu/healthwise/alice.html

Site(s) visited (URL): _____

List at least three strategies for preventing drunk driving:

Name _____ Section _____ Date _____

Nicotine Dependence: Are You Hooked?

Answer each question in the list below, giving yourself the appropriate points. Completing the smoking journal on the reverse may help you answer these questions more accurately.

		0 points	**1 point**	**2 points**
____	1. How soon after you wake up do you smoke your first cigarette?	After 30 minutes	Within 30 minutes	—
____	2. Do you find it difficult to refrain from smoking in places where it is forbidden, such as the library, theater, doctor's office?	No	Yes	—
____	3. Which of all the cigarettes you smoke in a day is the most satisfying?	Any other than the first one in the morning	The first one in the morning	—
____	4. How many cigarettes a day do you smoke?	1–15	16–25	26+
____	5. Do you smoke more during the morning than during the rest of the day?	No	Yes	—
____	6. Do you smoke when you are so ill that you are in bed most of the day?	No	Yes	—
____	7. Does the brand you smoke have a low, medium, or high nicotine content?	Low	Medium	High
____	8. How often do you inhale the smoke?	Never	Sometimes	Always

____ Total

Scoring

More than 6 points—very dependent

Less than 6 points—low to moderate dependence

(over)

Insel/Roth, *Core Concepts in Health*, Eighth Edition. © 1998 Mayfield Publishing Company. Chapter 11

Insel et al., *Core Concepts in Health*, Brief Eighth Edition. © 1998 Mayfield Publishing Company. Chapter 8

Smoking Journal

| Date _____ | | | | Day | M | TU | W | TH | F | SA | SU |

Time of day	N	R	Where were you?	What else were you doing?	Did someone else influence you?	Emotions and feelings?	Thoughts and concerns?

N = Number of cigarettes   R = Rating (0–3) of how much you wanted cigarette

QUIZ SOURCE: American Lung Association: Fagerstom Test.

Name _____ Section _____ Date _____

WELLNESS WORKSHEET 43

For Smokers Only: Why Do You Smoke?

Although smoking cigarettes is physiologically addicting, people smoke for reasons other than nicotine craving. What kind of smoker are you? Knowing what your motivations and satisfactions are can ultimately help you quit. This test is designed to provide you with a score on each of six factors that describe many people's smoking. Read the statements and then answer how *often* you feel this way when you smoke cigarettes. Be sure to answer each question.

		Always	Frequently	Occasionally	Seldom	Never
A.	I smoke cigarettes in order to keep myself from slowing down.	5	4	3	2	1
B.	Handling a cigarette is part of the enjoyment of smoking it.	5	4	3	2	1
C.	Smoking cigarettes is pleasant and relaxing.	5	4	3	2	1
D.	I light up a cigarette when I feel angry about something.	5	4	3	2	1
E.	When I have run out of cigarettes I find it almost unbearable until I can get them.	5	4	3	2	1
F.	I smoke cigarettes automatically without even being aware of it.	5	4	3	2	1
G.	I smoke cigarettes to stimulate me, to perk myself up.	5	4	3	2	1
H.	Part of the enjoyment of smoking a cigarette comes from the steps I take to light up.	5	4	3	2	1
I.	I find cigarettes pleasurable.	5	4	3	2	1
J.	When I feel uncomfortable or upset about something, I light up a cigarette.	5	4	3	2	1
K.	I am very much aware of the fact when I am not smoking a cigarette.	5	4	3	2	1
L.	I light up a cigarette without realizing I still have one burning in the ashtray.	5	4	3	2	1
M.	I smoke cigarettes to give me a "lift."	5	4	3	2	1
N.	When I smoke a cigarette, part of the enjoyment is watching the smoke as I exhale it.	5	4	3	2	1
O.	I want a cigarette most when I am comfortable and relaxed.	5	4	3	2	1
P.	When I feel "blue" or want to take my mind off cares and worries, I smoke cigarettes.	5	4	3	2	1
Q.	I get a real gnawing hunger for a cigarette when I haven't smoked for a while.	5	4	3	2	1
R.	I've found a cigarette in my mouth and didn't remember putting it there.	5	4	3	2	1

How to Score

1. Enter the numbers you have circled to the smoking questions in the scoring chart, putting the number you have circled to question A over line A, to question B over line B, and so on.

(over)

Insel/Roth, *Core Concepts in Health*, Eighth Edition. © 1998 Mayfield Publishing Company. Chapter 11
Insel et al., *Core Concepts in Health*, Brief Eighth Edition. © 1998 Mayfield Publishing Company. Chapter 8

2. Total the 3 scores on each line to get your totals. For example, the sum of your scores over lines A, G, and M gives you your score on *Stimulation*—lines B, H, and N give the score on *Handling,* etc.

Scoring Chart   Totals

_____ + _____ + _____ = _____
      A   G   M   Stimulation

_____ + _____ + _____ = _____
      B   H   N   Handling

_____ + _____ + _____ = _____
      C   I   O   Pleasurable relaxation

_____ + _____ + _____ = _____
      D   J   P   Crutch: Tension reduction

_____ + _____ + _____ = _____
      E   K   Q   Craving: strong physiological or psychological addiction

_____ + _____ + _____ = _____
      F   L   R   Habit

What Your Scores Mean

Scores can vary from 3 to 15. Any score 11 and above is *high;* any score 7 and below is *low.* The higher your score, the more important a particular factor is in your smoking and the more useful the discussion of that factor can be in your attempt to quit.

Stimulation If you score high on this factor, it means that you are stimulated by cigarettes—you feel that they help wake you up, organize your energies, and keep you going. Try substituting a brisk walk or moderate exercise whenever you feel the urge to smoke.

Handling A high score suggests you gain satisfaction from handling a cigarette. Try doodling or toying with a pen, pencil, or other small object.

Accentuation of Pleasure—Pleasurable Relaxation A high score on this factor suggests that you receive pleasure from smoking. Try substituting other pleasant situations or events such as social or physical activities.

Reduction of Negative Feelings, or "Crutch" A high score on this factor means you use cigarettes as a kind of crutch in moments of stress or discomfort. Physical exertion or social activity may serve as useful substitutes for cigarettes. Refer back to Chapter 2 for other strategies for dealing with stress.

Craving or Strong Addiction A high score on this factor indicates that you have a strong psychological craving for cigarettes. "Cold turkey" is probably your best approach to quitting. It may be helpful for you to smoke more than usual for a day or two, so that your taste for cigarettes is spoiled, and then isolate yourself completely from cigarettes until the craving is gone.

Habit A high score on this factor indicates that you smoke out of habit, not because smoking gives you satisfaction. Being aware of every cigarette you smoke and cutting down gradually may be effective quitting strategies for you.

Summary

Quitting smoking isn't easy. It usually means giving up something pleasurable that has a definite place in your life. In the end, of course, it's worth it. Now that you have some ideas about why you smoke, read the Behavior Change Strategy at the end of the chapter for a plan that will help you quit.

SOURCE: *Why Do You Smoke?* U.S. Department of Health and Human Services. Public Health Service. National Institutes of Health. NIH Pub. No 90-1822.

WELLNESS WORKSHEET 44

For Nonsmokers

List three things you might say to someone in asking him or her not to smoke in your presence. How would you defend your right to breathe smoke-free air?

1. _____

_____

2. _____

_____

3. _____

_____

List three situations where you recall being exposed to cigarette smoking. For each, describe what you might have done to avoid the situation.

1. _____

_____

2. _____

_____

3. _____

_____

If you've never smoked . . . Why do you think you never started smoking?

Did you have exposure to smokers (friends or family members) as you were growing up? How did this affect your decision not to smoke?

(over)

Insel/Roth, *Core Concepts in Health,* Eighth Edition. © 1998 Mayfield Publishing Company. Chapter 11
Insel et al., *Core Concepts in Health,* Brief Eighth Edition. © 1998 Mayfield Publishing Company. Chapter 8

What kinds of things do you think make people start smoking?

If you're an ex-smoker . . . How and why did you quit?

Can you offer any advice for the smoker who wants to quit?

INTERNET ACTIVITY

The World Wide Web provides many opportunities to become more involved in health issues that confront the United States, including tobacco use. Research ways to become an online tobacco activist. Visit the Web sites sponsored by the organizations listed below and/or do a search for additional tobacco-related sites.

    Action on Smoking and Health: http://ash.org

    Tobacco BBS: http://tobacco.org

    Smokescreen Tobacco Central Network: http://www.Smokescreen.org/

Site(s) visited (URL): _____

What opportunities for involvement did you discover? Do you think you are more likely to participate in online activist activities than activities that require personal contact? Why or why not?

WELLNESS WORKSHEET 45

Analyzing Advertisements

You can become more aware of the power that advertising can have by critically evaluating an ad. Choose a print ad for some type of tobacco product and answer the following questions. (Under regulations proposed in 1997, tobacco advertising may be severely restricted; if this occurs, complete this exercise using an ad for an alcoholic beverage.)

What is the verbal message of the ad? What does it say exactly? Are there direct references to the product?

Are certain words given unique treatment—larger or special type or a different color? Are there any plays on words or puns? How do these affect the message of the ad?

Are there any special offers or bargains such as savings coupons or merchandise offers?

How is the mandatory health warning handled in the ad?

What is the visual message of the ad? What images and symbols does it convey?

Is a famous person being used to sell the product? If so, how does this influence the effect the ad has on you?

(over)

Insel/Roth, *Core Concepts in Health,* Eighth Edition. © 1998 Mayfield Publishing Company. Chapter 11
Insel et al., *Core Concepts in Health,* Brief Eighth Edition. © 1998 Mayfield Publishing Company. Chapter 8

Who appears in the ad? Do they reflect American society or the tobacco (or alcohol) users in our society in terms of gender, ethnicity, age, and socioeconomic status? Who do you think is being targeted by the ad?

What does the ad convey about the people who use the product—in terms of their characteristics or lifestyle? (Examples of messages might include fun, success, independence, popularity, slimness, rebellion, wealth, sophistication, and relaxation.) What does the ad seem to promise to users of tobacco (or alcohol)?

How is sexuality portrayed? Is sexuality being used in any way to sell the product?

Think of the ad as a story. What story does it tell?

What is left unsaid by the ad? Will using the product transform a tobacco (or alcohol) user's life in the ways the ad suggests? What effects aren't portrayed in the ad?

SOURCE: Adapted from Teays, W. 1996. *Second Thoughts: Critical Thinking from a Multicultural Perspective.* Mountain View, Calif.: Mayfield.

Name _____ Section _____ Date _____

WELLNESS WORKSHEET 46

How's Your Diet?

- For each question, circle the plus (+) or minus (–) scores(s) that best reflects your diet. If you circle more than one score, average them by adding the scores and dividing by the number of scores you circled.
- For your final score, add your plus scores separately from your minus scores, then subtract your total minus scores from your total plus scores.
- Keep the quiz as incentive. Take it again in a few months to see if your habits have improved.

1. How many times a week do you eat red meat? (Include beef, lamb, pork, veal.)
   (a) 0   +4   (d) 5 or 6   –4
   (b) 1 or 2   +2   (e) More than 6   –5
   (c) 3 or 4   –2

2. How many ounces of red meat constitute your normal portion? (Hint: 3 ounces, cooked, is approximately the size of a deck of cards.)
   (a) 3 ounces   +2   (c) 5 ounces   –2
   (b) 4 ounces   +1   (d) 6 or more ounces   –3

3. What kind of red meat do you usually choose?
   (a) Loin or round cuts only   +2
   (b) 80% lean   +1
   (c) Ribs, T-bone   –4
   (d) Hot dogs, bacon, bologna   –5

4. How many times a week do you eat seafood? (Omit fried dishes; include shellfish like shrimp and lobster.)
   (a) 2 or more   +4   (c) Less than 1   0
   (b) 1   +2   (d) Never   –3

5. How many ounces of poultry or seafood do you eat for a serving? (Do not count fried items.)
   (a) 3 ounces   +2   (c) 5 ounces   –2
   (b) 4 ounces   +1   (d) 6 or more ounces   –3

6. Do you remove the skin from poultry?
   (a) Yes   +2   (c) No   –3
   (b) Don't eat poultry   0

7. How many times a week do you eat at least one half-cup serving of legumes? (Include beans like soybeans, navy, kidney, garbanzo, baked beans, lentils.)
   (a) 3 or more   +4   (c) Less than 1   0
   (b) 1 or 2   +2   (d) Never eat legumes   –1

8. What kind of milk do you drink?
   (a) Skim or 1%   +3   (c) 2%   –3
   (b) Don't drink milk   0   (d) Whole   –4

9. What kind of cheese do you usually eat?
   (a) Fat-free   +2
   (b) Lowfat (5 grams fat or less per ounce)   +1
   (c) Don't eat cheese   0
   (d) Whole milk cheese   –4

10. How many servings of lowfat, high-calcium foods do you eat daily? (One cup of yogurt or milk, 2 ounces of cheese, or one cup chopped broccoli, kale, or greens count as a serving.)
    (a) 3 or more   +4
    (b) 1 or 2   +2
    (c) 0   –3

11. What kind of bread do you eat most often?
    (a) 100% whole wheat   +4
    (b) Whole grain   +2
    (c) White, "wheat," Italian or French   0
    (d) Croissant or biscuit   –4

12. Which is part of your most typical breakfast?
    (a) High-fiber cereal and fruit   +4
    (b) Bagel or toast   +1
    (c) Don't eat breakfast   –2
    (d) Danish, pastry, or doughnut   –3

13. What kind of sauce or topping is usually on the pasta you eat?
    (a) Vegetables tossed lightly with olive oil   +3
    (b) Tomato or marinara sauce   +2
    (c) Meat sauce   –3
    (d) Alfredo or cream sauce   –4

14. Which would you be most likely to order at a Chinese restaurant?
    (a) Chicken with steamed vegetables over white rice   +3
    (b) Cold sesame noodles   –1
    (c) Twice-fried pork   –4

15. Which would you be most likely to choose as toppings for pizza?
    (a) Vegetables (e.g., broccoli, peppers)   +3
    (b) Plain cheese   0
    (c) Extra cheese   –3
    (d) Sausage and pepperoni   –4

(over)

Insel/Roth, *Core Concepts in Health,* Eighth Edition. © 1998 Mayfield Publishing Company. Chapter 12
Insel et al., *Core Concepts in Health,* Brief Eighth Edition. © 1998 Mayfield Publishing Company. Chapter 9

16. What is the most typical snack for you?
    (a) Fresh fruit   +4
    (b) Lowfat yogurt   +3
    (c) Pretzels   +1
    (d) Potato chips   −3
    (e) Candy bar   −3

17. How many half-cup servings of a high vitamin C fruit or vegetable do you eat daily? (Include citrus fruit and juices, kiwi, papaya, strawberries, broccoli, peppers, potatoes, tomatoes.)
    (a) 2 or more   +3
    (b) 1   +1
    (c) None   −3

18. How many half-cup servings of a high vitamin A fruit or vegetable do you eat daily? (Include apricots, cantaloupe, mango, broccoli, carrots, greens, spinach, sweet potato, winter squash.)
    (a) 2 or more   +3
    (b) 1   +1
    (c) None   −3

19. What kind of salad dressing do you most often choose?
    (a) Fat-free or lowfat   +3
    (b) Lemon juice or herb vinegar +3
    (c) Olive or canola oil-based   +1
    (d) Creamy or cheese-based   −3

20. What do you usually spread on bread, rolls, or bagels?
    (a) Nothing   +1
    (b) Jam, jelly, or honey   −1
    (c) Light butter or light margarine −2
    (d) Margarine   −3
    (e) Butter   −4

21. What spread do you usually choose for sandwiches?
    (a) Nothing   +3
    (b) Mustard   +2
    (c) Light mayonnaise   −1
    (d) Mayonnaise, margarine, or butter −3

22. Which frozen dessert do you usually choose?
    (a) Don't eat frozen desserts +3
    (b) Fat-free frozen yogurt   +1
    (c) Sorbet or sherbet   +1
    (d) Light ice cream   −2
    (e) Ice cream   −4

23. How many cups of caffeinated beverages (e.g., coffee, tea, or soda) do you usually drink in a typical day?
    (a) None   +2
    (b) 1 to 2   0
    (c) 3 or 4   −1
    (d) 5 or more −4

24. How many total cups of fluid do you drink in a typical day? (Include water, juice, milk.)
    (a) 8 or more   +3
    (b) 6 to 7   +2
    (c) 4 or 5   +1
    (d) Less than 4 −1

25. What kind of cereal do you eat?
    (a) High-fiber cereals such as bran flakes   +3
    (b) Low-fiber, low-sugar cereals, such as puffed rice, corn flakes, Corn Chex, or Cheerios.   0
    (c) Sugary, low-fiber cereals, like Frosted Flakes, or fruit-flavored cereals   −2
    (d) Regular (high-fat) granola   −3

26. How many times a week do you eat fried foods?
    (a) never   +4
    (b) 2 or less   0
    (c) 3 or more −3

27. How many times a week do you eat cancer-fighting cruciferous vegetables? (Include broccoli, cauliflower, brussels sprouts, cabbage, kale, bok choy, cooking greens, turnips, rutabaga.)
    (a) 3 or more +4
    (b) 1 to 2   +2
    (c) Rarely   −4

Score: _____ − _____ = _____
     (total of + answers)   (total of − answers)

Scoring
   65–82:   Excellent
   42–64:   Very good
   28–41:   Good
 −16–27:   Fair
Below −16:   Get help!

SOURCE: Copyright © 1993, CSPI. Adapted from Nutrition Action Healthletter (1875 Connecticut Ave., N.W., Suite 300, Washington, DC 20009–5728. $24 for 10 issues).

Name _____ Section _____ Date _____

WELLNESS WORKSHEET 47

Your Daily Diet versus the Food Guide Pyramid

To evaluate your daily diet for its nutritional value, you must first keep a record of everything you eat on a given day. Use the chart below to record all foods and beverages you consume; fill in the requested categories of information for all meals and snacks. Break down each food item you eat into its component parts (for example, a turkey sandwich should be listed as 2 slices of bread, 3 oz. of turkey, 1 t. mayonnaise, 1 t. mustard, 1 leaf of iceberg lettuce, one-half large tomato, etc.). You can complete the first two columns during the day; the remainder can be completed at the end of the day using information from your text.

Food	Portion size	Food group (see Food Guide Pyramid)	Number of servings* (see Food Guide Pyramid)

* Your portion sizes may be smaller or larger than the serving sizes given by the Food Guide Pyramid. List the actual number of servings contained in the foods you eat.

(over)

Insel/Roth, *Core Concepts in Health*, Eighth Edition. © 1998 Mayfield Publishing Company. Chapter 12
Insel et al., *Core Concepts in Health*, Brief Eighth Edition. © 1998 Mayfield Publishing Company. Chapter 9

Add up the total number of servings from each of the food groups listed on the Food Guide Pyramid and complete the following chart. Refer to your text for the recommended number of servings.

Food group	Recommended # of servings	# of servings consumed
Breads, cereals, rice, and pasta		
Vegetables		
Fruits		
Meat, poultry, fish, dry beans, eggs, and nuts		
Milk, yogurt, and cheese		

How does your daily diet rate when compared to the recommendations contained in the Food Guide Pyramid? Does this comparison indicate that you should increase or decrease your consumption of any particular group?

Using readily available foods that you like, create a sample daily diet that meets all the requirements of the Food Guide Pyramid.

WELLNESS WORKSHEET 48

Informed Food Choices

Part I. Using Food Labels

Choose three food items to evaluate. You might want to select three similar items, such as regular, lowfat, and nonfat salad dressing, or three very different items. Record the information from their food labels in the table below. How do the items you chose compare?

Food Items			
Serving size			
Total calories			
Total fat—grams			
—% Daily Value			
Saturated fat—grams			
—% Daily Value			
Cholesterol—milligrams			
—% Daily Value			
Sodium—milligrams			
—% Daily Value			
Carbohydrates (total)—grams			
—% Daily Value			
Dietary fiber—grams			
—% Daily Value			
Sugars—grams			
Protein—grams			
Vitamin A—% Daily Value			
Vitamin C—% Daily Value			
Calcium—% Daily Value			
Iron—% Daily Value			

Part II. Evaluating Fast Food

Use the information from Appendix A, Nutritional Content of Popular Items from Fast-Food Restaurants, to complete the chart on the next page for the last fast-food meal you ate. Add up your totals for the meal. Compare the values for fat, protein, carbohydrate, cholesterol, and sodium content for each food item and for the meal as a whole with the levels suggested by the Dietary Guidelines for Americans. Calculate the percent of total calories derived from fat, saturated fat, protein, and carbohydrate using the formulas given.

(over)

Insel/Roth, *Core Concepts in Health*, Eighth Edition. © 1998 Mayfield Publishing Company. Chapter 12
Insel et al., *Core Concepts in Health*, Brief Eighth Edition. © 1998 Mayfield Publishing Company. Chapter 9

If you haven't recently been to one of the restaurants included in the appendix, fill in the chart for any sample meal you might eat. If some of the food items you selected don't appear in Appendix A, ask for a nutrition information brochure when you visit the restaurant, or check out the online fast-food information at http://www.olen.com/food/

Food Items

	Dietary Guidelines							Total**
Serving size (g)		g	g	g	g	g	g	g
Calories								
Total fat*		g	g	g	g	g	g	g
	≤30%	%	%	%	%	%	%	%
Saturated fat*		g	g	g	g	g	g	g
	<10%	%	%	%	%	%	%	%
Protein*		g	g	g	g	g	g	g
	15%	%	%	%	%	%	%	%
Carbohydrate*		g	g	g	g	g	g	g
	≥55%	%	%	%	%	%	%	%
Cholesterol***	100 mg	mg	mg	mg	mg	mg	mg	mg
Sodium***	800 mg	mg	mg	mg	mg	mg	mg	mg

*To calculate the percent of total calories from each food energy source (fat, carbohydrate, protein), use the following formula:

$$\frac{(\text{number of grams of energy source}) \times (\text{number of calories per gram of energy source})}{(\text{total calories in serving of food item})}$$

(Note: fat and saturated fat provide 9 calories per gram; protein and carbohydrate provide 4 calories per gram.) For example, the percent of total calories from protein in a 150-calorie dish containing 10 grams of protein is:

$$\frac{(10 \text{ grams of protein}) \times (4 \text{ calories per gram})}{(150 \text{ calories})} = \frac{40}{150} = .27 \text{ or } 27\% \text{ of total calories from protein}$$

** For the Total column, add up the total grams of fat, carbohydrate, and protein contained in your sample meal and calculate the percentages based on the total calories in the meal. For cholesterol and sodium values, add up the total number of milligrams.

*** Recommended daily limits of cholesterol and sodium are divided by 3 here to give an approximate recommended limit for a single meal.

Name _____ Section _____ Date _____

WELLNESS WORKSHEET 49

Diabetes and Osteoporosis: Are You at Risk?

Part I. Diabetes Risk Assessment

This simple questionnaire can help you determine if you are among the 8 million Americans with diabetes who are currently undiagnosed. If the results indicate that you are at risk, don't panic or self-diagnose yourself. Only about 10% of people in the "at risk" category actually turn out to have the disease. However, if you are in the "at risk" category, you might want to speak with your physician about getting tested for diabetes.

Select the column that corresponds to your current age and answer the questions.

I am 20–44 years of age.	**I am 45–64 years of age.**	**I am 65+ years of age.**
My weight is equal to or above that listed in the weight chart. ____Yes ____ No	My weight is equal to or above that listed in the weight chart. ____Yes ____ No	My weight is equal to or above that listed in the weight chart. ____Yes ____ No
I get little or no exercise during a usual day. ____Yes ____ No	I get little or no exercise during a usual day. ____Yes ____ No	My mother, father, sister, or brother had diabetes. ____Yes ____ No
		I delivered a baby weighing over 9 lbs. ____Yes ____ No
If you answered yes to *both* questions, you are at risk!	If you answered yes to *either* question, you are at risk!	If you answered yes to *any* question, you are at risk!

	Women			Men	
Height		Weight	Height		Weight
Ft	In	lbs	Ft	In	lbs
4	9	134	5	1	157
4	10	137	5	2	160
4	11	140	5	3	162
5	0	143	5	4	165
5	1	146	5	5	168
5	2	150	5	6	172
5	3	154	5	7	175
5	4	157	5	8	179
5	5	161	5	9	182
5	6	164	5	10	186
5	7	168	5	11	190
5	8	172	6	0	194
5	9	175	6	1	199
5	10	179	6	2	203
5	11	182	6	3	209

Height is without shoes and weight is without clothes.

The chart shows weights which are 20% heavier than what is recommended for women and men with a medium frame (according to the Society of Actuaries and Association of Life Insurance Medical Directors of America: *Build Study,* 1979). If your weight is above the amount for your height, you may be at risk for developing diabetes.

For more information about diabetes—or to take an online diabetes risk assessment—contact the American Diabetes Association (160 Duke St., Alexandria, VA 22314; 800-342-2383; http://www.diabetes.org).

(over)

Insel/Roth, *Core Concepts in Health,* Eighth Edition. © 1998 Mayfield Publishing Company. Chapter 12
Insel et al., *Core Concepts in Health,* Brief Eighth Edition. © 1998 Mayfield Publishing Company. Chapter 9

Part II. Osteoporosis Risk Assessment
Complete the following questionnaire to determine your risk for developing osteoporosis.

Yes   No

_____ _____ 1. Do you have a small, thin frame?

_____ _____ 2. Do you have a family history of osteoporosis?

_____ _____ 3. Are you a postmenopausal woman?

_____ _____ 4. Have you had an early or surgically induced menopause?

_____ _____ 5. Have you been taking excessive thyroid medication or high doses of cortisone-like drugs for asthma, arthritis, or other disease?

_____ _____ 6. Is your diet low in dairy products and other sources of calcium?

_____ _____ 7. Are you physically inactive?

_____ _____ 8. Do you smoke cigarettes or drink alcohol in excess?

The more times you answer "yes," the greater your risk for developing osteoporosis. See your physician, or contact the National Osteoporosis Foundation for more information (1150 17th St., N.W., Suite 500, Washington DC, 20036; 202-223-2226; http://www.nof.org).

INTERNET ACTIVITY

Use the World Wide Web to find out more about diabetes or osteoporosis. Visit one of the Web sites on this worksheet or use a search engine to locate a related site. Describe the site and the types of information and services it provides. Is there information on risk factors, prevention, and treatment? Recent research findings? Help for finding a support group or a specialist? Was there anything you wanted to know about diabetes or osteoporosis that was not dealt with at the site you visited?

Site(s) visited (URL):_____

Description:

SOURCES: Part I adapted from *Diabetes Care,* Volume 18, Number 3, pp. 382–386, March 1995. Used with permission of The American Diabetes Association. Part II reprinted with permission from the National Osteoporosis Foundation, Washington, D.C. (202) 223-2226.

Name _____ Section _____ Date _____

WELLNESS WORKSHEET 50

Food Safety Quiz

Fill in the correct answer to each question.

_____ 1. Mayonnaise and foods prepared with mayonnaise, such as potato salad, are common sources of foodborne illness. True or false?

_____ 2. After handling raw meat, poultry, or fish, you should wash your hands with warm water and soap. True or false?

_____ 3. The warmest safe temperature for refrigerated food is 50°F (10°C). True or false?

_____ 4. Canned foods can be kept indefinitely. True or false?

_____ 5. Food that is contaminated with a foodborne pathogen often looks and smells completely normal. True or false?

_____ 6. Approximately what percentage of raw ground poultry sold in stores is contaminated with *Salmonella?*
   a. 15%
   b. 30%
   c. 50%

_____ 7. Which of the following is a safe method for defrosting meat or poultry?
   a. setting it on the kitchen counter
   b. placing it in the refrigerator
   c. microwaving it

_____ 8. How long is it safe to store ground meat in the refrigerator prior to using it?
   a. 1–2 days
   b. 3–4 days
   c. 1 week

_____ 9. The best place to store milk and eggs in the refrigerator is
   a. the door
   b. an inside shelf

_____ 10. In the event of a power failure, how long will food in the refrigerator last?
   a. 1–2 hours
   b. 4–6 hours
   c. 10–12 hours

_____ 11. How long will an opened package of hotdogs keep in the refrigerator?
   a. 3–4 days
   b. 1 week
   c. 2 weeks

_____ 12. A whole roasted turkey or chicken should be cooked to what temperature?
   a. 140° F
   b. 160° F
   c. 180° F

_____ 13. If you use a sponge to clean up kitchen counters or cutting boards that have come in contact with raw meat, poultry, or fish, you should
   a. rinse the sponge with water and let it dry completely
   b. place the sponge in the dishwasher

_____ 14. What is the maximum amount of time that perishable food can safely be left out of the refrigerator?
   a. 30 minutes
   b. 2 hours
   c. 5 hours

(over)

Insel/Roth, *Core Concepts in Health,* Eighth Edition. © 1998 Mayfield Publishing Company. Chapter 12
Insel et al., *Core Concepts in Health,* Brief Eighth Edition. © 1998 Mayfield Publishing Company. Chapter 9

_____ 15. When you eat out, it's safe to order your hamburger cooked
   a. rare
   b. medium
   c. well-done

Answers

1. False. Store-bought mayonnaise is usually made from pasteurized eggs and contains other ingredients such as salt and lemon juice that can slow the growth of foodborne pathogens. Eating foods made with homemade mayonnaise made with raw eggs is riskier.
2. True. Just wiping hands on a towel or rinsing them under tap water, even hot tap water, will not remove foodborne pathogens. Hands should be washed in soapy water for at least 20 seconds.
3. False. Food safety experts recommend a temperature of 41°F (5°C) or less. Consumers should use a thermometer to check their refrigerator's temperature and adjust the control dial as needed.
4. False. Canned foods last a long time, but not forever. Two years is a safe limit for most foods, but highly acidic foods such as tomatoes should be used within one year.
5. True. Most food that is contaminated has no strange odor or visible mold.
6. c. About 20% of broiler chickens and 10% of raw ground beef is also contaminated.
7. b or c. Foodborne pathogens can multiply quickly at room temperature. If using the microwave, cook foods immediately after thawing.
8. a. Ground meats should be refrigerated and then cooked or frozen within 1–2 days of purchase.
9. b. Foods in the door don't stay as cold as foods stored in other parts of the refrigerator. Highly perishable food items should be stored on an inside shelf, which stays colder.
10. b. Without power, the refrigerator will keep food cool about 4–6 hours, depending on the temperature of the room. Placing blocks of ice on refrigerator shelves can help keep food cooler for a longer period of time.
11. b. An opened package will keep about a week, an unopened package for about 2 weeks. Lunch meats perish more quickly and should be used within 3–5 days of being opened.
12. c. Use a meat thermometer in several spots to check that the food is heated all the way through.
13. b. It's best to avoid using sponges to clean up potentially contaminated surfaces. If you do use sponges, place them in the dishwasher daily.
14. b. Foodborne pathogens multiply rapidly at room temperature. If you are going on a picnic, pack food in insulated carriers with cold packs.
15. c. It's safest to order your hamburger well-done—cooked until it is no longer red in the middle and the juices run clear.

Scoring

Give yourself 1 point for each correct answer to questions 1–5 and 2 points for each correct answer to questions 6–15.

Score	Rating
25	Excellent
20–24	Very good
12–19	Need improvement
11 or below	Reexamine your food handling practices

SOURCES: Food and Drug Administration. 1996. Can your kitchen pass the food safety test? Reprint from *FDA Consumer Magazine.* FDA pub. no. 96-1229. What's your food safety IQ? 1996. *Environmental Nutrition,* June. USDA Food Safety and Inspection Service. 1995. *A Quick Consumer Guide to Safe Food Handling.* Home and Garden Bulletin No. 248.

WELLNESS WORKSHEET 51

Do You Need to Increase Your Level of Physical Activity?

Part I. Medical Clearance

In general, if you are under thirty-five, have no physical complaints, and have had a medical checkup within the past two years, it is probably safe for you to begin an exercise program at your current level of physical activity and gradually increase it. To determine whether you need to consult your physician, read through the following list of statements and check any that are true for you.

_____ I am not feeling well.

_____ I have a specific health concern.

_____ I am over 20% above my desirable weight and much of the excess is body fat.

_____ I have been sedentary for a long time.

_____ I have a history of some type of cardiovascular disease.

_____ I can't walk more than two miles.

_____ I have one or more of the following symptoms after exertion:

    _____ Chest pain

    _____ Dizziness or faintness

    _____ Gastrointestinal upset

    _____ Difficulty breathing

    _____ Shortness of breath for more than 10 minutes after exertion

    _____ Lingering fatigue and difficulty in sleeping

_____ I am 35 or older and have a history of coronary heart disease risk factors:

    _____ Diabetes

    _____ Hypertension

    _____ High blood cholesterol levels

    _____ Cigarette smoking

    _____ A blood relative who had a heart attack before age 60

If you checked one or more of these statements, you should consult your physician before beginning any type of exercise program.

Part II. Calculate Your Activity Index

1. Frequency: How often do you exercise?

If you exercise:	Your frequency score is:
Less than 1 time a week	0
1 time a week	1
2 times a week	2
3 times a week	3
4 times a week	4
5 or more times a week	5

(over)

Insel/Roth, *Core Concepts in Health,* Eighth Edition. © 1998 Mayfield Publishing Company. Chapter 13
Insel et al., *Core Concepts in Health,* Brief Eighth Edition. © 1998 Mayfield Publishing Company. Chapter 10

2. Duration: How long do you exercise?

If each session continues for:	Your duration score is:
Less than 5 minutes	0
5 to 14 minutes	1
15 to 29 minutes	2
30 to 44 minutes	3
45 to 59 minutes	4
60 minutes or more	5

3. Intensity: How hard do you exercise?

If exercise results in:	Your intensity score is:
No change in pulse from resting level	0
Little change in pulse from resting level (slow walking, bowling, yoga)	1
Slight increase in pulse and breathing (table tennis, active golf with no golf cart)	2
Moderate increase in pulse and breathing (leisurely bicycling, easy continuous swimming, rapid walking)	3
Intermittent heavy breathing and sweating (tennis singles, basketball, squash)	4
Sustained heavy breathing and sweating (jogging, cross-country skiing, rope skipping)	5

To calculate your activity index, multiply your three scores:

Frequency _____ × Duration _____ × Intensity _____ = Activity index _____

To assess your activity index, refer to the following table:

If your activity index is:	Your estimated level of activity is:
Less than 15	Sedentary
15–24	Low active
25–40	Moderate active
41–60	Active
Over 60	High active

If your activity level is in one of the lower categories, review the components of your score (frequency, duration, intensity) to see how you can raise your score. Add to your current exercise program or devise a new one.

SOURCE: Kusinitz, I., and M. Fine. 1995. *Your Guide to Getting Fit,* 3d ed. Mountain View, Calif.: Mayfield.

Name _____ Section _____ Date _____

 WELLNESS WORKSHEET 52

Evaluating Your Fitness Level

Once you've decided whether you should obtain medical clearance before making a change in your exercise program, the next step is to assess your current level of physical fitness. The tests presented here will allow you to make a relatively simple assessment of cardiorespiratory endurance, muscular endurance, and flexibility. The results from these tests can help show you what to focus on as you develop a fitness program.

I. Cardiorespiratory Endurance
1.5-Mile Run-Walk Test

(Don't attempt this test unless you have completed at least six weeks of some type of conditioning activity and, if indicated by Wellness Worksheet 51, have obtained medical clearance.) Before beginning this test, warm up with some walking, easy jogging, and stretching exercises.

1. Ask someone with a stopwatch, clock, or watch with a second hand to time you.
2. Take the test on a running track or course that is flat and provides measurements of up to 1.5 miles. Cover the distance as fast as possible, at a pace that is comfortable for you. You can run or walk the entire distance or use some combination of running and walking.
3. Note the time it takes you to complete the 1.5-mile distance.
   Your time: ____ : ____ (minutes:seconds)
4. Cool down by walking or jogging slowly for about 5 minutes.
5. Determine the rating for your score by consulting the table below. If you are unable to complete the entire 1.5 miles, consider yourself very poor in CRE.

Standards for the 1.5-Mile Run-Walk Test (minutes:seconds)

Women	Superior	Excellent	Good	Fair	Poor	Very Poor
Age: 18–29	11:00 or less	11:15–12:45	13:00–14:15	14:30–15:45	16:00–17:30	17:45 or more
30–39	11:45 or less	12:00–13:30	13:45–15:15	15:30–16:30	16:45–18:45	19:00 or more
40–49	12:45 or less	13:00–14:30	14:45–16:30	16:45–18:30	18:45–20:45	21:00 or more
50–59	14:15 or less	14:30–16:30	16:45–18:30	18:45–20:30	20:45–23:00	23:15 or more
60 and over	14:00 or less	14:15–17:15	17:30–20:15	20:30–22:45	23:00–24:45	25:00 or more

Men						
Age: 18–29	9:15 or less	9:30–10:30	10:45–11:45	12:00–12:45	13:00–14:00	14:15 or more
30–39	9:45 or less	10:00–11:00	11:15–12:15	12:30–13:30	13:45–14:45	15:00 or more
40–49	10:00 or less	10:15–11:45	12:00–13:00	13:25–14:15	14:30–16:00	16:25 or more
50–59	10:45 or less	11:00–12:45	13:00–14:15	14:30–15:45	16:00–17:45	18:00 or more
60 and over	11:15 or less	11:30–13:45	14:00–15:45	16:00–17:45	18:00–20:45	21:00 or more

SOURCES: Formula for maximal oxygen consumption taken from McArdle, W. D., F. I. Katch, and V. L. Katch. 1991. *Exercise Physiology: Energy, Nutrition, and Human Performance.* Philadelphia: Lea & Febiger, pp. 225–226. Ratings based on norms from the Cooper Institute for Aerobics Research, Dallas, Texas, *The Physical Fitness Specialist Manual*, revised 1993. Used with permission.

(over)

12-Minute Wheelchair Performance Test

1. Warm up before taking the test. Take the test on a track or course that is flat and provides exact distance measurements in miles.
2. Travel at a steady pace, as fast as possible without undue fatigue, for the entire 12 minutes. Cool down after the test is over.
3. Record the distance you traveled in miles, using a decimal figure.
   Distance traveled: _____ miles

Ratings for the 12-Minute Wheelchair Performance Test

Distance (miles)	Fitness Level
Below 0.63	Poor
0.63–0.86	Below average
0.87–1.35	Fair
1.36–1.59	Good
Above 1.59	Excellent

SOURCE: Franklin, B. A., et al. 1990. Field test estimation of maximal oxygen consumption in wheelchair users. *Archives of Physical Medicine and Rehabilitation* 71: 574–578.

II. Muscular Strength and Endurance
The 60-Second Sit-Up Test

Do not take this test if you suffer from low-back pain. To prepare, try a few sit-ups to get used to the proper technique and warm up your abdominal muscles.

1. Lie flat on your back on the floor with knees bent, feet flat on the floor, and your fingers interlocked behind your neck. Your partner should hold your ankles firmly so that your feet stay on the floor as you do the sit-ups.
2. When someone signals you to begin, raise your head and chest off the floor until your elbows touch your knees or thighs, then return to the starting position. Keep your neck neutral. Do not force your neck forward, and stop if you feel any pain.
3. Perform as many sit-ups as you can in 60 seconds.
   Number of sit-ups: _____

Ratings for the 60-Second Sit-Up Test

Men		Very Poor	Poor	Fair	Good	Excellent	Superior
Age:	Under 20	Below 36	36–40	41–46	47–50	51–61	Above 61
	20–29	Below 33	33–37	38–41	42–46	47–54	Above 54
	30–39	Below 30	30–34	35–38	39–42	43–51	Above 51
	40–49	Below 24	24–28	29–33	34–38	39–47	Above 47
	50–59	Below 19	19–23	24–27	28–34	35–43	Above 43
	60 and over	Below 15	15–18	19–21	22–29	30–38	Above 38

Number of Sit-Ups

(over)

Number of Sit-Ups

Women		Very Poor	Poor	Fair	Good	Excellent	Superior
Age:	Under 20	Below 28	28–31	32–35	36–45	46–54	Above 54
	20–29	Below 27	27–31	32–37	38–43	44–50	Above 50
	30–39	Below 20	20–24	25–28	29–34	35–41	Above 41
	40–49	Below 14	14–19	20–23	24–28	29–37	Above 37
	50–59	Below 10	10–13	14–19	20–23	24–29	Above 29
	60 and over	Below 3	3–5	6–10	11–16	17–27	Above 27

SOURCE: Based on norms from the Cooper Institute for Aerobics Research, Dallas, Texas, *The Physical Fitness Specialist Manual,* revised 1993. Used with permission.

The Push-Up Test

In this test, you will perform either standard push-ups or modified push-ups, in which you support yourself with your knees. The Cooper Institute developed the ratings for this test with men performing push-ups and women performing modified push-ups.

1. *For push-ups:* Start in the push-up position with your body supported by your hands and feet. *For modified push-ups:* Start in the modified push-up position with your body supported by your hands and knees. *For both positions,* your arms and your back should be straight and your fingers pointed forward.
2. Lower your chest to the floor with your back straight, then return to the starting position.
3. Perform as many push-ups or modified push-ups as you can without stopping.
   Number of push-ups: _____ or number of modified push-ups: _____

Ratings for the Push-Up and Modified Push-Up Tests

Number of Push-Ups

Men		Very Poor	Poor	Fair	Good	Excellent	Superior
Age:	18–29	Below 22	22–28	29–36	37–46	47–61	Above 61
	30–39	Below 17	17–23	24–29	30–38	39–51	Above 51
	40–49	Below 11	11–17	18–23	24–29	30–39	Above 39
	50–59	Below 9	9–12	13–18	19–24	25–38	Above 38
	60 and over	Below 6	6–9	10–17	18–22	23–27	Above 27

Number of Modified Push-Ups

Women		Very Poor	Poor	Fair	Good	Excellent	Superior
Age:	18–29	Below 17	17–22	23–29	30–35	36–44	Above 44
	30–39	Below 11	11–18	19–23	24–30	31–38	Above 38
	40–49	Below 6	6–12	13–17	18–23	24–32	Above 32
	50–59	Below 6	6–11	12–16	17–20	21–27	Above 27
	60 and over	Below 2	2–4	5–11	12–14	15–19	Above 19

SOURCE: Based on norms from the Cooper Institute for Aerobics Research, Dallas, Texas, *The Physical Fitness Specialist Manual,* revised 1993. Used with permission.

(over)

III. Flexibility
Sit-and-Reach Test

Warm up your muscles with some low-intensity activity such as walking or easy jogging.

1. Place a firm box on the floor against a wall. Tape a ruler on the box so that the 6-inch mark is on line with the near edge of the box and the 12-inch mark is farthest from you at the wall end of the box.
2. Remove your shoes, and sit facing the flexibility box with your knees fully extended and your feet about 4 inches apart. Your feet should be flat against the box.
3. Reach as far forward as you can, with palms down and one hand placed on top of the other. Hold the position of maximum reach for 1–2 seconds. Keep your knees locked at all times.
4. Repeat the stretch two times. Your score is the most distant point reached with the fingertips of both hands on the third trial, measured to the nearest quarter of an inch.

   Score of third trial: _____ in.

Ratings for Sit-and-Reach Test

		Rating/Score (in.)*			
Men		*Very Poor*	*Poor*	*Moderate*	*High*	*Very High*
Age:	15–19	Below 5.25	5.25–6.75	7.00–8.75	9.00–10.75	Above 10.75
	20–29	Below 5.50	5.50–7.00	7.25–8.75	9.00–11.00	Above 11.00
	30–39	Below 4.75	4.75–6.50	6.75–8.50	8.75–10.25	Above 10.25
	40–49	Below 2.75	2.75–5.00	5.25–6.75	7.00–9.25	Above 9.25
	50–59	Below 2.00	2.00–5.00	5.25–6.50	6.75–9.25	Above 9.25
	60 and over	Below 1.75	1.75–3.25	3.50–5.25	5.50–8.50	Above 8.50
Women						
Age:	15–19	Below 7.25	7.25–8.75	9.00–10.50	10.75–12.25	Above 12.25
	20–29	Below 6.75	6.75–8.50	8.75–10.00	10.25–11.50	Above 11.50
	30–39	Below 6.50	6.50–8.00	8.25–9.50	9.75–11.50	Above 11.50
	40–49	Below 5.50	5.50–7.25	7.50–8.75	9.00–10.50	Above 10.50
	50–59	Below 5.50	5.50–7.25	7.50–8.50	8.75–10.75	Above 10.75
	60 and over	Below 4.75	4.75–6.00	6.25–7.75	8.00–9.25	Above 9.25

*Footline is set at 6 inches.

SOURCE: Adapted from Fitness Canada. 1986. *CSTF Operations Manual,* 3d ed. Ottowa: Fitness and Amateur Sport. The Canadian Standardized Test of Fitness was developed by, and is reproduced with permission of Fitness Canada, Government of Canada.

A Summary of Your Fitness

Components and Tests	Rating

Cardiorespiratory endurance
   1.5-mile run-walk test or
   12-minute wheelchair performance test	

Muscular strength and endurance
   60-second sit-up test
   Push-up or modified push-up test	

Flexibility Sit-and-reach	

Use the information in this summary chart to help choose activities for your fitness program.

WELLNESS WORKSHEET 53

What's Your Excuse for Not Exercising?

Some of these statements apply to people who have not yet started to exercise, and some apply to people who started but quit. Circle the letter next to any statement that applies to you.

(C)   1. I am afraid that exercise will make me look silly.

(A)   2. I exercised for a while, then stopped when I went on vacation.

(P)   3. I exercised, but it never felt easy or pleasant.

(K)   4. I will exercise sometime—when I can get my outfit color-coordinated.

(R)   5. I quit because I didn't seem to be improving.

(S)   6. People often laughed at me when I expressed enthusiasm for exercise.

(P)   7. Exercise hurt: My muscles were always sore.

(W)   8. I only exercised because my spouse/physician wanted me to.

(T)   9. I don't have time.

(M) 10. I think exercise will increase my appetite, and I will put on weight.

(P) 11. I get very tired and/or short of breath when I exercise.

(R) 12. I felt I would never be as thin (or agile) as the others in the class/group.

(W) 13. I simply disliked every type of exercise I tried.

(M) 14. I am afraid I might have a heart attack.

(T) 15. I will exercise when I move closer to my work/when the kids grow up/when I get a different job.

(S) 16. I don't like to exercise alone.

(K) 17. I can't decide which exercise to try.

(A) 18. I used to exercise but stopped when I got sick.

(M) 19. (For women): I am afraid of developing large muscles.

(S) 20. I didn't like the people in the class/group.

(C) 21. I think exercise is a fad, and people will laugh at me for being fashionable.

(T) 22. I would exercise if the day were an hour longer.

(R) 23. I quit because I never achieved my goals.

(P) 24. I tried exercising and was sore for a week.

(A) 25. I was just getting started when some relatives came to stay or the weather turned bad or something.

Add up the number of times you circled each letter, and write the totals here:

T: _____ W: _____ R: _____ S: _____ P: _____ K: _____ M: _____ A: _____ C:_____

If you scored points in any category, read the appropriate section.

(over)

Insel/Roth, *Core Concepts in Health,* Eighth Edition. © 1998 Mayfield Publishing Company. Chapter 13
Insel et al., *Core Concepts in Health,* Brief Eighth Edition. © 1998 Mayfield Publishing Company. Chapter 10

T: Time Management

If you have trouble finding time for exercise, you are not alone. Try getting up earlier in the morning for a walk, doubling up on your activities (read the paper or watch TV while you ride your exercise bicycle), or hiring a gardener or babysitter to free up time. Make a commitment to exercise, and find the time.

A: You Accidentally Quit

If your exercise program gets thrown off by illness, travel, or houseguests, make a commitment to get back on track as soon as your routine returns to normal. Most travel destinations will have exercise opportunities; if nothing else, walk up and down hotel corridors and stairs.

M: Myths

Exercise need not provoke heart attacks, increase weight, or make women look masculine. For solid information about exercise, refer to your textbook.

S: Social Support

Find a group of people you enjoy exercising with and arrange your schedule to include them. Social support will make your exercise program more enjoyable and easier to stick with.

R: Realistic Expectations

You may be expecting either too much or too little of yourself, and it is interfering with the reality of what you can actually do. Most people can improve steadily in both strength and stamina if they begin gradually and stick to their program consistently. However, few people can run marathons in their second week, and some should never think of running marathons at all. Set realistic goals for yourself and your program.

W: Something's Seriously Wrong

You should exercise for yourself, not for others. Make fitness fun by finding activities you enjoy. Try "play" activities such as inline skating, surfing, skiing, dancing, or basketball. Try walking while listening to books on tape or music. Activities such as housework, yardwork, and cleaning the car can also be part of your fitness program if they raise your heart rate.

K: Who Are You Trying to Kid?

Your commitment is wobbly at best. Review the benefits of exercise, and find yourself someone to buddy up with in order to start an exercise program.

P: Physical Problems

If you experienced chest pains or extreme shortness of breath, talk with your physician. Otherwise, start with low-intensity exercise, and increase the intensity of your program very gradually. Expect some minor muscle aches and tiredness, but don't exercise so vigorously that you feel terrible for days. Warm up, cool down, and do plenty of stretching exercises.

C: You Feel Conspicuous

Try exercising at home or joining a health club or class with people who are in the same shape you are. Take up walking and bring your dog along.

SOURCE: Adapted by permission from *Fresh Start: The Stanford Medical School Health & Fitness Program* by the Stanford Center for Research in Disease Prevention (KQED Books 1996).

Name _____ Section _____ Date _____

WELLNESS WORKSHEET 54

Personal Fitness Program Plan and Contract

A. I, _____, am contracting with myself to follow a physical fitness
        (name)

program to work toward the following goals:

1. _____

2. _____

3. _____

4. _____

5. _____

B. My program plan is as follows:

Activities	Components (Check ✓)					Intensity	Duration	Frequency (Check ✓)						
	CRE	MS	ME	F	BC			M	Tu	W	Th	F	Sa	Su

C. My program will begin on _____. My program includes the following schedule of
                              (date)

minigoals. For each step in my program, I will give myself the reward listed.

_____   _____   _____
        (minigoal 1)   (date)   (reward)

_____   _____   _____
        (minigoal 2)   (date)   (reward)

_____   _____   _____
        (minigoal 3)   (date)   (reward)

D. My program will include the addition of physical activity to my daily routine (such as walking to class):

1. _____   4. _____

2. _____   5. _____

3. _____   6. _____

(over)

Insel/Roth, *Core Concepts in Health*, Eighth Edition. © 1998 Mayfield Publishing Company. Chapter 13
Insel et al., *Core Concepts in Health*, Brief Eighth Edition. © 1998 Mayfield Publishing Company. Chapter 10

E. I will use the following tools to monitor my program and my progress toward my goals:

_____
(list any charts, graphs, or journals you plan to use)

_____

I sign this contract as an indication of my personal commitment to reach my goal.

_____   _____
(your signature)   (date)

I have recruited a helper who will witness my contract and _____

_____
(list any way your helper will participate in your program)

_____   _____
(witness's signature)   (date)

INTERNET ACTIVITY

Select one of the activities you've chosen for your fitness program; use a search engine to locate Web sites that relate to the activity.

How many total sites did the search engine locate relating to your activity? _____

Find at least two helpful sites and provide a brief description of each. Look for information that will help you safely enjoy the activity you've chosen.

Activity: _____

Site 1 (URL): _____

Description:

Site 2 (URL): _____

Description:

About how many sites did you have to visit before locating two useful ones? _____

Describe the overall list of sites. Were they mostly commercial, sponsored by people or businesses selling products related to the activity, or were there many sites sponsored by individuals and organizations?

WELLNESS WORKSHEET 60

Facts About the Cardiovascular System

Review your knowledge of the cardiovascular system by filling in the blanks and answering the questions below. Refer to your textbook if necessary.

1. The cardiovascular system consists of the _____ and the blood vessels. Name and describe the three major types of blood vessels.

    a. _____

    _____

    b. _____

    _____

    c. _____

    _____

2. Name and define the two separate circulatory systems.

    a. _____

    _____

    b. _____

    _____

3. What changes occur when blood reaches the lungs?

    _____

    _____

4. About how much blood does each person have? _____

    How often does the total volume of blood circulate through the system? _____

5. How is the heart supplied with oxygenated blood?

    _____

    _____

6. Describe the electrical system that controls the heartbeat.

    _____

    _____

    _____

    _____

(over)

7. Trace the path of blood through the cardiorespiratory system by filling in the blanks.

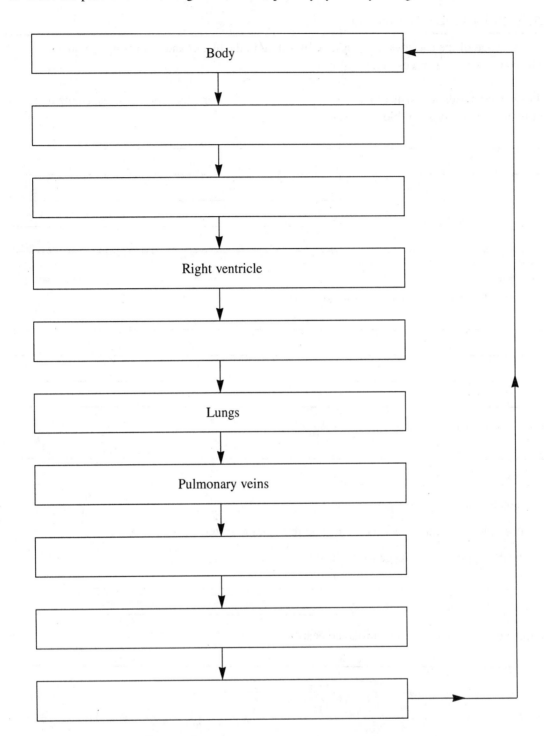

Body

[blank]

[blank]

Right ventricle

[blank]

Lungs

Pulmonary veins

[blank]

[blank]

[blank]

Name _____ Section _____ Date _____

WELLNESS WORKSHEET 61

Are You at Risk for Cardiovascular Disease?

Your chances of suffering an early heart attack or stroke depend on a variety of factors, many of which are under your control. To help identify your risk factors, circle the response for each risk category that best describes you.

1. Gender

   0 Female
   2 Male

2. Heredity

   0 Neither parent suffered a heart attack or stroke before age 60.
   3 One parent suffered a heart attack or stroke before age 60.
   7 Both parents suffered a heart attack or stroke before age 60.

3. Smoking

   0   Never smoked
   1   Quit more than 2 years ago
   2   Quit less than 2 years ago
   8   Smoke less than 1/2 pack per day
   13 Smoke more than 1/2 pack per day
   15 Smoke more than 1 pack per day

4. Environmental Tobacco Smoke

   0 Do not live or work with smokers
   2 Exposed to ETS at work
   3 Live with smoker
   4 Both live and work with smokers

5. Blood Pressure

   The average of the last three readings:
   0   130/80 or below
   1   131/81 to 140/85
   5   141/86 to 150/90
   9   151/91 to 170/100
   13 Above 170/100

6. Total Cholesterol

   The average of the last three readings:
   0 Lower than 190
   1 190 to 210
   2 Don't know
   3 211 to 240
   4 241 to 270
   5 271 to 300
   6 Over 300

7. HDL Cholesterol

   The average of the last three readings:
   0   Over 65 mg/dl
   1   55 to 65
   2   Don't know HDL
   3   45 to 54
   5   35 to 44
   7   25 to 34
   12 Lower than 25

8. Exercise

   0 Aerobic exercise three times per week
   1 Aerobic exercise once or twice per week
   2 Occasional exercise less than once per week
   7 Rarely exercise

9. Diabetes

   0   No personal or family history
   2   One parent with diabetes
   6   Two parents with diabetes
   9   Non–insulin-dependent diabetes
   13 Insulin-dependent diabetes

10. Weight

    0 Near ideal weight
    1 6 pounds or less above ideal weight
    3 7 to 19 pounds above ideal weight
    5 20 to 40 pounds above ideal weight
    7 More than 40 pounds above ideal weight

11. Stress

    0 Relaxed most of the time
    1 Occasional stress and anger
    2 Frequently stressed and angry
    3 Usually stressed and angry

(over)

Insel/Roth, *Core Concepts in Health,* Eighth Edition. © 1998 Mayfield Publishing Company. Chapter 15
Insel et al., *Core Concepts in Health,* Brief Eighth Edition. © 1998 Mayfield Publishing Company. Chapter 12

Scoring

Total your risk factor points. Refer to the list below to get an approximate rating of your risk of suffering an early heart attack or stroke.

Score	Estimated Risk
Less than 20	Low risk
20–29	Moderate risk
30–45	High risk
Over 45	Extremely high risk

Whatever your score, examine your responses carefully to identify your CVD risk factors. Consider planning a behavior change strategy to lower your risk by changing your lifestyle.

INTERNET ACTIVITY

Use the World Wide Web to learn more about one of the controllable risk factors for cardiovascular disease. Choose one of the risk factors from the quiz in this worksheet—preferably one for which you have a high score. Find out more about the risk factor by visiting the American Heart Association's online Heart and Stroke A–Z Guide (http://www.americanheart.org) or by doing a Web search.

Risk factor: _____

Site(s) visited (URL): _____

What did you learn about the risk factor? Did you identify any strategies you can apply to your daily life? Any changes you can make in your current behavior to control or lessen the risk factor?

WELLNESS WORKSHEET 62

Facts About Cardiovascular Disease

Review your knowledge of CVD by filling in the blanks and answering the questions below. Refer to your textbook if necessary.

1. What are the four main risk factors for cardiovascular disease?

   a. _____   c. _____

   b. _____   d. _____

2. List six additional factors that may increase risk for cardiovascular disease.

   a. _____   d. _____

   b. _____   e. _____

   c. _____   f. _____

3. Name the two main forms of cholesterol and describe their function.

   a. _____

   _____

   b. _____

   _____

4. Describe the difference between systolic and diastolic pressure. Give normal and high ranges for each.

   _____

   _____

   _____

   Why is hypertension dangerous? _____

   _____

   List two treatments for hypertension.

   a. _____

   b. _____

5. What is atherosclerosis? How do plaques form, and why are they dangerous?

   _____

   _____

(over)

Insel/Roth, *Core Concepts in Health,* Eighth Edition. © 1998 Mayfield Publishing Company. Chapter 15
Insel et al., *Core Concepts in Health,* Brief Eighth Edition. © 1998 Mayfield Publishing Company. Chapter 12

_____

_____

6. What is a heart attack? _____

   _____

   What are angina pectoris and arrhythmia, and how do they relate to heart attacks?

   _____

   _____

   _____

   What are three early signals of a heart attack?

   a. _____   c. _____

   b. _____

   List and describe two surgical procedures performed to prevent heart attacks.

   a. _____

   _____

   b. _____

   _____

7. List and describe the three major types of strokes.

   a. _____

   _____

   b. _____

   _____

   c. _____

   _____

   List three warning signs of a stroke.

   a. _____   c. _____

   b. _____

8. What are the two main causes of heart disease in children?

   a. _____

   b. _____

WELLNESS WORKSHEET 63

Hostility Quiz and Log

Current research indicates that there are three aspects of hostility that are particularly harmful to health: cynicism (a mistrusting attitude regarding other people's motives), anger (an emotional response to other people's "unacceptable" behavior), and aggression (behaviors in response to negative emotions such as anger and irritation). To get an idea of how hostile you are, check any of the following statements that are true for you.

_____ 1. Stuck in a long line at the express checkout in the grocery store, I often count the number of items the people in front of me have to see if anyone is over the limit.

_____ 2. I am often irritated by other people's incompetence.

_____ 3. If a cashier gives me the wrong change, I assume he or she is probably trying to cheat me.

_____ 4. I've been so angry at someone that I've thrown things or slammed a door.

_____ 5. If someone is late, I plan the angry words I'm going to say.

_____ 6. I tend to remember irritating incidents and get mad all over again.

_____ 7. If someone cuts me off in traffic, I honk my horn, flash my lights, pound the steering wheel, or shout.

_____ 8. Little annoyances have a way of adding up during the day, leaving me frustrated and impatient.

_____ 9. If the person who cuts my hair trims off more than I want, I fume about it for days afterward.

_____ 10. When I get into an argument, I feel my jaw clench and my pulse and breathing rate climb.

_____ 11. If someone mistreats me, I look for an opportunity to pay them back, just for the principle of the thing.

_____ 12. I find myself getting annoyed at little things my spouse or significant other does that get under my skin.

Add up the number of items you checked. A score of 3 or less indicates a generally cool head. A score between 4 and 8 indicates that your level of hostility could be raising your risk of heart disease. A score of 9 or more indicates a hot head—a level of cynicism, anger, and aggression high enough to endanger both heart health and interpersonal relationships.

If you are a hot head, try keeping a log of your hostile responses to people and situations (see over). Familiarize yourself with the patterns of thinking that lead to hostile feelings, and try to head them off before they develop into full-blown anger. If you feel your anger starting to build, ask yourself the following questions:

1. *Is this really important enough to get angry about?* For example, is having to wait an extra 5 minutes for a late bus so important that you should stew about it for the entire 5-minute ride?

2. *Are you really justified in getting angry?* Is the person in front of you really driving slowly, or are you trying to speed?

3. *Is getting angry going to make any real difference in this situation?* Will slamming the door really help your friend find the concert tickets he misplaced?

If you answer "yes" to all three questions, then you should calmly but assertively ask for what you want. A "no" to any question means that you should try to diffuse your anger. Reason with yourself, distract your mind with another activity, or try one of the techniques for meditation or deep breathing described in Chapter 2 in your text.

(over)

Insel/Roth, *Core Concepts in Health*, Eighth Edition. © 1998 Mayfield Publishing Company. Chapter 15
Insel et al., *Core Concepts in Health*, Brief Eighth Edition. © 1998 Mayfield Publishing Company. Chapter 12

Hostility Journal

Date _____

Time	Location	What happened?	What were you thinking?	What were you feeling?	What did you do?

WELLNESS WORKSHEET 67

Facts About Pathogens and How They Cause Disease

Part I. Pathogens

Familiarize yourself with different types of pathogens by completing the chart below. Refer to your textbook if necessary.

	Description and Examples	Diseases Caused	Possible Treatments
Bacteria			
Viruses			
Fungi			
Protozoa			
Parasitic worms			

(over)

Insel/Roth, *Core Concepts in Health,* Eighth Edition. © 1998 Mayfield Publishing Company. Chapter 17
Insel et al., *Core Concepts in Health,* Brief Eighth Edition. © 1998 Mayfield Publishing Company. Chapter 13

Part II. Chain of Infection

Fill in the steps in the chain of infection, and write a brief description of each step. List at least two ways that the chain can be broken at each step.

Chain of Infection   **Description**

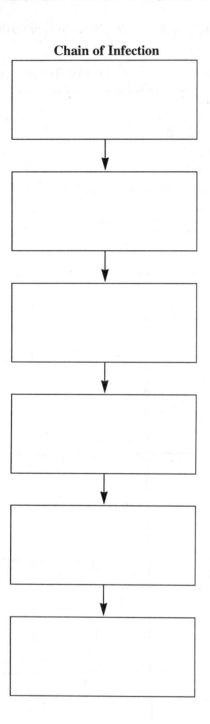

Name _____ Section _____ Date _____

Review your knowledge of infection and immunity by answering the questions below. Refer to your textbook if necessary

1. List and describe three of the body's physical or chemical barriers against infection.

   a. _____

   b. _____

   c. _____

2. What general type of cells carry out the immune response? _____

   _____

   Where are these immune defenders produced? _____

   _____

   Describe each of the following types of cells and explain their role in the immune response.

   Neutrophils _____

   _____

   Macrophages _____

   _____

   Natural killer cells _____

   _____

   Helper T cells _____

   _____

   Killer T cells _____

   _____

   Suppressor T cells _____

   _____

   B cells _____

   _____

   Memory T and B cells _____

   _____

   _____

(over)

Insel/Roth, *Core Concepts in Health,* Eighth Edition. © 1998 Mayfield Publishing Company. Chapter 17
Insel et al., *Core Concepts in Health,* Brief Eighth Edition. © 1998 Mayfield Publishing Company. Chapter 13

3. What are antibodies? What is their role in the immune response?

_____

_____

_____

4. How do the body's defenders recognize an enemy? What is an antigen?

_____

_____

_____

5. What is the inflammatory response? _____

_____

_____

6. Briefly describe the four phases of the immune response.

a._____

_____

b._____

_____

c._____

_____

d._____

_____

7. What is immunity? When and how does it occur? _____

_____

_____

_____

8. When is an infected person contagious? _____

_____

_____

9. What is a vaccine? _____

_____

What are the two types of immunity that a vaccine can confer?

a._____

b._____

10. What is an allergic reaction, and how does it occur? _____

_____

_____

WELLNESS WORKSHEET 69

Checklist for Avoiding Infection

The best thing you can do to prevent an infection is to limit your exposure to pathogens. The next best thing is to keep your immune system as strong as possible. Read through the following list of statements and check whether each is mostly true or mostly false for you.

True   False

Exposure to Pathogens

____   ____   I receive drinking water from a clean supply.

____   ____   The area in which I live has adequate sewage treatment.

____   ____   I frequently wash my hands with soap and warm water.

____   ____   I avoid close contact with people who are infectious with diseases transmitted via the respiratory route (e.g., influenza, chicken pox, and tuberculosis).

____   ____   I do not inject drugs.

When Outdoors

____   ____   When hiking or camping, I do not drink water from streams, rivers, or lakes without first purifying it.

____   ____   I avoid contact with ticks, rodents, and other disease carriers.

____   ____   When hiking in the woods or playing in a yard in an area where Lyme disease has been reported, I take appropriate precautions:

____   Wear long pants, a long-sleeved shirt, and closed shoes.

____   Tuck my shirt into my pants and my pants into my socks, shoes, or boots.

____   Wear light-colored, tightly woven fabrics.

____   Wear a hat.

____   Stay near the center of trails.

____   Check myself periodically for ticks.

____   Shower and shampoo after each outing.

____   Wash clothes and check equipment after each outing

____   Use an insect repellent containing DEET on my skin and/or a spray containing permethrin on my clothing.

____   ____   If I discover a tick attached to my skin, I remove it immediately in an appropriate

manner (fill in): _____

_____

_____

_____

(over)

Insel/Roth, *Core Concepts in Health,* Eighth Edition. © 1998 Mayfield Publishing Company. Chapter 17
Insel et al., *Core Concepts in Health,* Brief Eighth Edition. © 1998 Mayfield Publishing Company. Chapter 13

True **False**

In a Sexual Relationship

____ ____ I am in a monogamous relationship with a mutually faithful, uninfected partner.

____ ____ I use condoms.

____ ____ I discuss STDs and prevention with new partners.

____ ____ I avoid engaging in high-risk behaviors with any person who might carry HIV.

In the Kitchen

____ ____ I wash my hands thoroughly with hot soapy water before and after handling food.

____ ____ I don't let groceries sit in a warm car.

____ ____ I avoid buying food in containers that leak, bulge, or are severely dented.

____ ____ I use separate cutting boards for meat and for foods that will be eaten raw.

____ ____ I thoroughly clean all equipment (cutting boards, counters, utensils) before and after use.

____ ____ I wash fresh fruits and vegetables carefully to remove all dirt.

____ ____ I cook all foods thoroughly, especially beef, poultry, fish, pork, and eggs.

____ ____ I store foods below 40°F.

____ ____ I do not leave cooked or refrigerated foods at room temperature for more than two hours.

____ ____ I thaw foods in the refrigerator or microwave.

____ ____ I use only pasteurized milk and juice.

____ ____ I avoid coughing or sneezing over foods, even when I'm healthy.

____ ____ I cover any cuts on my hands when handling food.

To Keep Your Immune System Healthy

____ ____ I eat a balanced diet, following the guidelines presented in the Food Guide Pyramid and the Dietary Guidelines for Americans.

____ ____ I maintain a healthy weight.

____ ____ I get enough sleep, 6–8 hours per night.

____ ____ I exercise regularly.

____ ____ I don't smoke.

____ ____ I have effective ways of coping with stress.

____ ____ I get all recommended immunizations and booster shots.

False answers indicate areas where you could change your behavior to help avoid infectious diseases. Consider creating a behavior change strategy for any statement you checked false.

WELLNESS WORKSHEET 70

Personal Infectious Disease and Allergy Record

Part I. Infectious Diseases

Place a check next to any of the following infectious diseases you have had. Where appropriate, list your age at the time of the infection and any special circumstances surrounding the time of the infection (e.g., your entire first grade class got the chicken pox; you got mononucleosis at a time of high stress) in the box provided. Circle any disease for which you have been vaccinated.

_____ Influenza	_____ Tetanus	_____ Pinworm
_____ Chicken pox	_____ Hepatitis A	_____ HIV infection
_____ Rubella (German measles)	_____ Hepatitis B or C	_____ Chlamydia
_____ Measles	_____ Lyme disease	_____ Gonorrhea
_____ Mumps	_____ Polio	_____ Genital warts (HPV)
_____ Strep throat	_____ Rabies	_____ Herpes
_____ Whooping cough (pertussis)	_____ Malaria	_____ Syphilis
_____ Diphtheria	_____ Cholera	_____ Trichomoniasis
_____ Rheumatic fever	_____ Yeast infection	_____ Pubic lice
_____ Scarlet fever	_____ Bladder infection	_____ Scabies
_____ Mononucleosis	_____ Athlete's foot	_____ Other: _____
_____ Pneumonia	_____ Jock itch	_____ Other: _____
_____ Tuberculosis	_____ Ringworm	_____ Other: _____

Disease	Age	Circumstances

(over)

Part II. Allergies

Put a check next to any substance to which you have had an allergic reaction; if appropriate, list the specific type of substance you are allergic to (cats, spider bites, nuts, etc.). Describe the type of reaction you had.

✔ Allergen	Specific Type(s)	Reaction(s)
Poison ivy or oak		
Animals		
Feathers		
Insect bites or stings		
Molds		
Dust mites		
Ragweed		
Pollen		
Foods		
Other:		

Describe any allergy tests you've undergone and any treatments you've received.

Name _____ Section _____ Date _____

WELLNESS WORKSHEET 71

Facts About Sexually Transmitted Diseases

Familiarize yourself with different types of sexually transmitted diseases by completing the chart below.

	Early symptoms	Potential long-term effects	Diagnosis and treatment
HIV infection			
Chlamydia			
Gonorrhea			
Pelvic inflammatory disease			
Genital warts			

(over)

Insel/Roth, *Core Concepts in Health*, Eighth Edition. © 1998 Mayfield Publishing Company. Chapter 18
Insel et al., *Core Concepts in Health*, Brief Eighth Edition. © 1998 Mayfield Publishing Company. Chapter 13

	Early symptoms	Potential long-term effects	Diagnosis and treatment
Genital herpes			
Hepatitis B			
Syphilis			

INTERNET ACTIVITY

Visit several of the sites listed in the For More Information section of Chapter 18 in your text (Chapter 13 in the brief version)—or do a Web search—to complete one of the following activities.

   1. Find information on STD prevention and safer sex. Look for strategies for talking with a sex partner, saying no to sex or drugs, or using a condom correctly.

   2. Find information about a recent development or advance in HIV incidence, treatment, prevention, or testing. Look for a site with news posted within the past month.

Site visited (URL): _____

Information available from site:

Name _____ Section _____ Date _____

WELLNESS WORKSHEET 72

Do Your Attitudes and Behaviors Put You at Risk for STDs?

Part I. Risk Assessment

All sexually transmitted diseases are preventable. You have control over the behaviors and attitudes that place you at risk for contracting STDs and for increasing their negative effects on your health. To identify your risk factors for STDs, read the following list of statements and identify whether they're true or false for you.

True   **False**

_____   _____   1. I have never been sexually active (If false, continue. If true, you are not at risk; respond to the remaining statements based on how you realistically believe you would act.)

_____   _____   2. I am in a mutually faithful relationship with an uninfected partner or am not currently sexually active. (If false, continue. If true, you are at minimal risk now; respond to the remaining statements according to your attitudes and past behaviors.)

_____   _____   3. I have only one sexual partner.

_____   _____   4. I always use a latex condom for each act of intercourse, even if I am fairly certain my partner has no infections.

_____   _____   5. I do not use oil-based lubricants with condoms.

_____   _____   6. I discuss STDs and prevention with new partners before having sex.

_____   _____   7. I do not use alcohol or another mood-altering drug in sexual situations.

_____   _____   8. I would tell my partner if I thought I had been exposed to an STD.

_____   _____   9. I am familiar with the signs and symptoms of STDs.

_____   _____   10. I regularly perform genital self-examination.

_____   _____   11. When I notice any sign or symptom of any STD, I consult my physician immediately.

_____   _____   12. I obtain screening for HIV and other STDs regularly. In addition (if female), I obtain yearly pelvic exams and Pap tests.

_____   _____   13. When diagnosed with an STD, I inform all recent partners.

_____   _____   14. When I have a sign or symptom of an STD that goes away on its own, I still consult my physician.

_____   _____   15. I do not use drugs prescribed for friends or partners or left over from other illnesses to treat STDs.

_____   _____   16. I do not share syringes or needles to inject drugs.

False answers indicate attitudes and behaviors that may put you at risk for contracting STDs or for suffering serious medical consequences from them.

(over)

Part II. Communication

1. List three ways to bring up the subject of STDs with a new partner. How would you ask whether or not he or she has been exposed to any STDs or engaged in any risky behaviors? (Remember that since many STDs can be asymptomatic it is important to know about past behaviors even if no STD was diagnosed.)

   a. _____

   _____

   b. _____

   _____

   c. _____

   _____

2. List three ways to bring up the subject of condom use with your partner. How might you convince someone who does not want to use a condom?

   a. _____

   _____

   b. _____

   _____

   c. _____

   _____

3. If you had had an STD in the past that you might possibly still pass on (e.g., herpes), how would you tell your partner(s)?

   _____

   _____

   _____

4. If you were diagnosed with an STD that you believe was given to you by your current partner, how would you begin a discussion of STDs with him or her?

   _____

   _____

Talking about STDs may be a bit awkward, but the temporary embarrassment of asking intimate questions is a small price to pay to avoid contracting or spreading disease.

Name _____ Section _____ Date _____

WELLNESS WORKSHEET 73

What Happens to Your Body as You Age?

Review your knowledge of the physical changes that accompany aging by filling in the chart below. Refer to your textbook if necessary.

	Changes
Skin	
Body fat	
Hearing	
Eyesight	
Taste and smell	
Hair	
Bones	
Muscles	

(over)

Insel/Roth, *Core Concepts in Health,* Eighth Edition. © 1998 Mayfield Publishing Company. Chapter 19
Insel et al., *Core Concepts in Health,* Brief Eighth Edition. © 1998 Mayfield Publishing Company. Chapter 14

	Changes
Teeth	
Heart	
Lungs	
Digestive system	
Kidneys	
Immune system	
Brain and nervous system	
Sexual organs and sexual response	

Name _____ Section _____ Date _____

WELLNESS WORKSHEET 74

Are You Prepared for Aging?

Assess Your Current Behaviors

Are you doing everything you can now to enhance the quality of your life as you age? Read through the following list of statements and check the answer that best describes your current behavior.

Yes   **No**

____   ____   I exercise regularly.

____   ____   I eat wisely.

                ____   I eat meals low in fat and high in complex carbohydrates (fresh fruits and vegetables, whole-grain cereals and breads, brown rice, pasta).

                ____   I avoid saturated fats and get protein from fish and skinless poultry.

                ____   I use nonfat or low-fat dairy products.

                ____   I consume the recommended amount of calcium.

                ____   I limit the amount of sodium I consume.

____   ____   My weight is in the recommended range.

____   ____   I drink alcohol in moderation, if at all.

____   ____   I don't smoke or use smokeless tobacco.

____   ____   I recognize the stressors in my life and take appropriate steps to control and deal with stress.

____   ____   I perform appropriate self-examinations.

____   ____   I have regular physical examinations that include appropriate screening tests.

____   ____   I participate in activities that keep my mind sharp and active.

Thinking About Aging

Have you thought seriously about the changes that aging can bring? To help you begin thinking now about your life as you grow older, answer the following questions.

1. What things come to mind when you think of an older person? Can you imagine those things applying to you? What do you think you will be like when you are 70 years old?

2. What do you most look forward to as you grow older?

(over)

Insel/Roth, *Core Concepts in Health*, Eighth Edition. © 1998 Mayfield Publishing Company. Chapter 19
Insel et al., *Core Concepts in Health*, Brief Eighth Edition. © 1998 Mayfield Publishing Company. Chapter 14

3. What do you most fear as you grow older?

4. How long would you like to keep working? What would you like to do after you retire? What hobbies or volunteer opportunities would you pursue?

5. Have you considered the loss of income that retirement often brings? What can you do now to help meet your economic needs in the future?

6. Older people often find themselves alone more frequently (due to the death of a spouse and/or close friends). Can you think of activities you enjoy doing alone?

7. If when you are older you are no longer able to care for yourself, what living and care arrangements would you prefer?

8. What would you do if your parents were no longer able to care for themselves?

9. List five positive and five negative things about aging.

Name _____ Section _____ Date _____

 WELLNESS WORKSHEET 75

Your Experiences and Attitudes About Death

Learning to accept and deal with death is a difficult but important part of life. Examine your past experiences and attitudes about death by answering the questions below. Circle the answer that best describes your experiences or attitudes and fill in the requested information.

1. Who died in your first personal involvement with death?

    a. Grandparent or great-grandparent
    b. Parent
    c. Brother or sister
    d. Other family member
    e. Friend or acquaintance
    f. Stranger
    g. Public figure
    h. Animal

2. To the best of your memory, at what age were you first aware of death?

    a. Under three
    b. Three to five
    c. Five to ten
    d. Ten or older

3. When you were a child, how was death talked about in your family?

    a. Openly
    b. With some sense of discomfort
    c. Only when necessary and then with an attempt to exclude the children
    d. As though it were a taboo subject
    e. Never recall any discussion

4. Which of the following best describes your childhood conceptions of death?

    a. Heaven and hell concept
    b. Afterlife
    c. Death as sleep
    d. Cessation of all physical and mental activity
    e. Mysterious and unknowable
    f. Something other than the above
    i. No conception
    h. Can't remember

5. Which of the following most influenced your present attitudes toward death?

    a. Death of someone close
    b. Specific reading
    c. Religious upbringing
    d. Introspection and meditation
    e. Ritual (e g., funerals)
    f. TV, radio, or motion pictures
    g. Longevity of my family
    h. My health or physical condition
    i. Other (specify): _____

    _____

6. To what extent do you believe in a life after death?

    a. Strongly believe in it
    b. Tend to believe in it
    c. Uncertain
    d. Tend to doubt it
    e. Convinced it does not exist

7. Regardless of your belief about life after death, what is your wish about it?

    a. I strongly wish there were a life after death.
    b. I am indifferent as to whether there is a life after death.
    c. I definitely prefer that there not be a life after death.

8. How often do you think about your own death?

    a. Very frequently (at least once a day)
    b. Frequently
    c. Occasionally
    d. Rarely (no more than once a year)
    e. Very rarely or never

9. If you could choose, when would you die?

    a. In youth
    b. In the middle prime of life
    c. Just after the prime of life
    d. In old age

(over)

10. When do you believe that, in fact, you will die?

    a. In youth
    b. In the middle prime of life
    c. Just after the prime of life
    d. In old age

11. Has there been a time in your life when you wanted to die?

    a. Yes, mainly because of great physical pain
    b. Yes, mainly because of great emotional pain
    c. Yes, mainly to escape an intolerable social or interpersonal situation
    d. Yes, mainly because of great embarrassment
    e. Yes, for a reason other than above
    f. No

12. What does death mean to you?

    a. The end; the final process of life
    b. The beginning of a life after death; a transition, a new beginning
    c. A joining of the spirit with a universal cosmic consciousness
    d. A kind of endless sleep; rest and peace
    e. Termination of this life but with survival of the spirit
    f. Don't know
    g. Other (specify): _____
       _____

13. What aspect of your own death is the most distasteful to you?

    a. I could no longer have any experience.
    b. I am afraid of what might happen to my body after death.
    c. I am uncertain as to what might happen to me if there is a life after death.
    d. I could no longer provide for my family.
    e. It would cause grief to my relatives and friends.
    f. All my plans and projects would come to an end.
    g. The process of dying might be painful.
    h. Other (specify): _____
       _____

14. In your opinion, at what age are people most afraid of death?

    a. Up to 12 years
    b. 13 to 19 years
    c. 20 to 29 years
    d. 30 to 39 years
    e. 40 to 49 years
    f. 50 to 59 years
    g. 60 to 69 years
    h. 70 years and over

15. When you think of your own death or when circumstances make you aware of your own mortality, how do you feel?

    a. Fearful
    b. Discouraged
    c. Depressed
    d. Purposeless
    e. Resolved, in relation to life
    f. Pleasure, in being alive
    g. Other (specify): _____
       _____

16. To what extent are you interested in having your image survive after your own death through your children, books, good works, etc.?

    a. Very interested
    b. Moderately interested
    c. Somewhat interested
    d. Not very interested
    e. Totally uninterested

17. If you had a choice, what kind of death would you prefer?

    a. Tragic, violent death
    b. Sudden but not violent death
    c. Quiet, dignified death
    d. Death in line of duty
    e. Death after a great achievement
    f. Suicide
    g. Homicide
    h. There is no "appropriate" kind
    i. Other (specify): _____
       _____

18. If it were possible, would you want to know the exact date on which you are going to die?

    a. Yes
    b. No

(over)

19. How important do you believe mourning and grief ritual (such as wakes and funerals) are for the survivors?

    a. Extremely important
    b. Somewhat important
    c. Undecided or don't know
    d. Not very important
    e. Not important at all

20. If it were entirely up to you, how would you like to have your body disposed of after you have died?

    a. Burial
    b. Cremation
    c. Donation to medical school or science
    d. I am indifferent

21. What kind of a funeral would you prefer?

    a. Formal, as large as possible
    b. Small, relatives and close friends only
    c. Whatever my survivors want
    d. None

22. How do you feel about "lying in state" in an open casket at your funeral?

    a. Approve
    b. Don't care one way or the other
    c. Disapprove
    d. Strongly disapprove

23. Who do you feel should be the one to tell you that you are dying?

    a. Physician
    b. Nurse
    c. Family member
    d. Close friend

24. Which aspect of yourself would you want to take time with if you knew you would die soon? Rate 1–10 for urgency, 1 being most urgent.

    a. Physical
    b. Emotional
    c. Activities and plans
    d. Spiritual
    e. Relationships
    f. Playful
    g. Financial and practical
    h. Other (specify): _____
    _____

25. List four things you would most like to learn, change, or do before you die. Number 1 through 4 in priority

    _____
    _____
    _____
    _____

26. Which rituals or activities do you feel may be helpful for survivors and their grief process? Mark V = Very helpful, M = Moderately helpful, Q = Questionable, N = Not helpful, D = Detrimental.

    a. Embalming, open casket
    b. Viewing body, not embalmed
    c. Memorial service
    d. Getting rid of photos and belongings
    e. Taking trip later
    f. Remembering dead on anniversary, holidays
    g. Talking about deceased a lot
    h. New social activities, dating
    i. Wearing black
    j. Taking a trip right away
    k. Restricting social activities
    l. Keeping belongings
    m. Moving, selling house (when not necessary)
    n. Joining widows' group
    o. Grieving alone
    p. Sharing grief with children
    q. Suggested activities not mentioned:
    _____
    _____
    _____
    _____

27. Most often, how do you feel you probably will die?

    a. Long illness
    b. Stroke or heart attack
    c. Auto crash
    d. War
    e. Violent encounter
    f. Other (specify): _____
    _____

(over)

28. What is your most vivid experience with death?
Age: _____
    a. Dream
    b. Experience with close person
    c. Animal
    d. Experience with stranger
    e. Story
    f. News story
    If your answer was (a), (c), or (f), briefly describe: _____
    _____

29. How is death talked about in your family at this time?
    a. Openly
    b. Some discomfort
    c. Only when necessary
    d. Excludes children
    e. Taboo
    f. Never recall talking
    g. Excludes dying person or survivor

30. At what age did you experience the most fear of death? _____
    Do you know what was on your mind then?
    _____

31. If you had a terminal illness, who would you want to talk with about your "difficult" feelings? (Number in preferential order):
    a. Spouse
    b. Close family member
    c. Physician
    d. Another patient
    e. Friend
    f. Nurse
    g. Therapist
    h. Clergy or spiritual friend
    i. Understanding third party

32. If a physician told you that an immediate family member was going to die, would you want them told?
    a. Yes
    b. No
    c. Depends

33. If your close friend was dying, felt depressed, and wanted to talk, how would you feel?
    a. Comfortable
    b. Embarrassed
    c. Distressed
    d. Willing
    e. Not sure
    f. Would visit less

34. When thinking of dying, I mostly fear (Rate H = High fear, M = Moderate fear, L = Low fear):
    a. Being alone
    b. Mentally disoriented
    c. Pain
    d. Disfigurement
    e. Dependence on others
    f. Loss of control over physical functions
    g. What happens at/after death
    h. Hospitalization for treatment
    i. Other (specify): _____
    _____

35. When notified of a funeral—not immediate family—I usually:
    a. Decline
    b. Hate to go
    c. Happy to go
    d. Attend if at all possible
    e. Dread going

36. The cause of death I'm most afraid of is:
    a. Accident
    b. Cancer
    c. Bomb
    d. Infection
    e. Nerve disease
    f. Heart failure
    g. Kidney failure
    h. Stroke
    i. Violence
    j. Other (specify): _____
    _____

SOURCE: From Edwin S. Shneidman, The Energy: You and Death questionnaire, *Psychology Today,* August 1970. Reprinted with permission from Psychology Today magazine.

Name _____ Section _____ Date _____

WELLNESS WORKSHEET 76

Planning for Death

Once you acknowledge the inevitability of death, you can plan for it and ease what might later be hard decisions for both your survivors and yourself. Some decisions can and should be made early so that an unexpected death is not made even more difficult for family and friends. Think about plans you can make for your own death by answering the questions below.

1. *Make a will.* You should make out a will when you reach the age of majority. It should include specific instructions about how to dispose of your property. List ten possessions in the space below and indicate whom they should go to in the event of your death.

List any money or investments you have (bank accounts, certificates of deposit, 401(k) accounts, etc.). Who should this money go to? How should it be divided?

If applicable, create some general guidelines for your executor regarding children or ongoing business investments.

(over)

2. *Decide what to do with your body.* Would you prefer your body to be embalmed or not, buried, cremated, given to medicine for research, or prepared for donating organs? What are the reasons for your choice? If you decide to donate organs, complete a Uniform Donor Card and carry it in your wallet.

3. *Plan a ceremony.* What type of ceremony would you prefer? If you choose to have a gravestone, what would you want it to say? If you have chosen cremation, what would you like done with the ashes?

4. *Choose where to die.* If death is not sudden and you have a choice, where would you prefer to spend your last days (home, hospital, hospice)? Consider the effects of your choice on you, your family, and your finances.

Name _____ Section _____ Date _____

WELLNESS WORKSHEET 77

Advance Medical Directives

You can obtain a standard advance directive for your state from a local hospital, a state health department, or the not-for-profit organization Choice in Dying (200 Varick St., New York, NY 10014; 212-366-5540). The state forms are not very specific, and you may increase the chance of a physician following your wishes if you provide more detailed instructions. The form shown below allows you to make specific choices about medical procedures under six different circumstances.

This form expresses my specific wishes regarding medical treatments in case illness prevents me from communicating them directly. My wishes apply both to the illness described and to any other situations that might develop. If a circumstance arises that my choices do not specifically address, my doctors and my agent should extrapolate from my choices below to the situation at hand. I understand that my wishes must be medically reasonable. Finally, all conclusions about my medical condition must be agreed to by my physician and appropriate consultants.

For each of the situations at right, check the boxes that indicate your wishes regarding treatment	Situation A If I am in a coma or persistent vegetative state and have no known hope of recovering awareness or higher mental functions:			Situation B If I am in a coma and have a small but uncertain chance of regaining awareness and higher mental functioning:			Situation C If I am aware but have brain damage that makes me unable to recognize people, to speak meaningfully, or to live independently, and I have a terminal illness:		
	I want	I do not want	I want a trial; if no clear improvement, stop treatment.	I want	I do not want	I want a trial; if no clear improvement, stop treatment.	I want	I do not want	I want a trial; if no clear improvement, stop treatment.
1. Cardiopulmonary resuscitation. The use of pressure on the chest, drugs, electric shocks, and artificial breathing to revive me if my heart stops.			■						■
2. Mechanical respiration. Breathing by machine, through a tube in the throat.									
3. Artificial feeding. Giving food and water through a tube inserted either in a vein, down the nose, or through a hole in the stomach.									
4. Major surgery. For example, removing the gallbladder or part of the intestine.			■						■
5. Kidney dialysis. Cleaning the blood by machine or by fluid passed through the abdomen.									
6. Chemotherapy. Drugs to fight cancer.									
7. Minor surgery. For example, removing part of an infected toe.			■			■			
8. Invasive diagnostic tests. For example, examining the stomach through a tube inserted down the throat.			■			■			
9. Transfusions of blood or blood components.									
10. Antibiotics. Drugs to fight infection.									
11. Simple diagnostic tests. For example, blood tests or X rays.			■			■			■
12. Pain medications, even if they dull consciousness and indirectly shorten my life.						■			

Insel/Roth, *Core Concepts in Health,* Eighth Edition. © 1998 Mayfield Publishing Company. Chapter 20
Insel et al., *Core Concepts in Health,* Brief Eighth Edition. © 1998 Mayfield Publishing Company. Chapter 14

(over)

For each of the situations at right, check the boxes that indicate your wishes regarding treatment.	Situation D — If I am aware but have brain damage that makes me unable to recognize people, to speak meaningfully, or to live independently, and I do not have a terminal illness:			Situation E — If I have an incurable chronic illness that causes physical suffering or minor mental disability and will ultimately cause death, and then I develop a life-threatening but reversible illness:			Situation F — If I am in my current state of health (describe briefly)_____ _____ _____ and then develop a life-threatening but reversible disease:		
	I want	I do not want	I want a trial; if no clear improvement, stop treatment.	I want	I do not want	I want a trial; if no clear improvement, stop treatment.	I want	I do not want	I want a trial; if no clear improvement, stop treatment.
1. Cardiopulmonary resuscitation. The use of pressure on the chest, drugs, electric shocks, and artificial breathing to revive me if my heart stops.			█						█
2. Mechanical respiration. Breathing by machine, through a tube in the throat.									
3. Artificial feeding. Giving food and water through a tube inserted either in a vein, down the nose, or through a hole in the stomach.									
4. Major surgery. For example, removing the gallbladder or part of the intestine.			█						█
5. Kidney dialysis. Cleaning the blood by machine or by fluid passed through the abdomen.									
6. Chemotherapy. Drugs to fight cancer.									
7. Minor surgery. For example, removing part of an infected toe.			█			█			█
8. Invasive diagnostic tests. For example, examining the stomach through a tube inserted down the throat.			█			█			█
9. Transfusions of blood or blood components.									
10. Antibiotics. Drugs to fight infection.									
11. Simple diagnostic tests. For example, blood tests or X rays.			█			█			█
12. Pain medications, even if they dull consciousness and indirectly shorten my life.			█						█

Signed: _____

Signature _____ Printed name

Address _____ Date

Witness: _____

Signature _____ Printed name

Address _____ Date

Witness: _____

Signature _____ Printed name

Address _____ Date

Name _____ Section _____ Date _____

WELLNESS WORKSHEET 78

Personal Health Profile

Complete the following personal health profile and keep it with Wellness Worksheet 70 (Personal Infectious Disease and Allergy Record) so that you have a compete record of your health status. Keep your profile up-to-date.

Age: _____   Height: _____   Weight: _____

Current Conditions or Diseases   **Treatments and Medications**

_____   _____
_____   _____
_____   _____
_____   _____
_____

Current Conditions or Diseases Common in Your

Family (see Wellness Worksheet 34)   **Ethnic Group**

_____   _____
_____   _____
_____   _____
_____   _____

Prescription Medication Information

Drug	Prescription No.	No. of Refills	Pharmacy Telephone
_____	_____	_____	_____
_____	_____	_____	_____
_____	_____	_____	_____
_____	_____	_____	_____

Health care provider:_____ _____

Pharmacy: _____ _____

(over)

Record of Medical Tests and Exams

Enter the date of your most recent test, exam, or vaccination.

Date	Test/Exam/Vaccination	Recommended Frequency
_____	Blood pressure check	Every 1–2 years
_____	Cholesterol measurement	Every 5 years for men 35–65 and women 45–85
_____	Screening for HIV infection and other STDs	Routinely for pregnant women and others at risk
_____	Tuberculosis test	Members of high-risk groups only
_____	Vision test	Every 2–3 years
_____	Fecal occult blood test	Every year for people over 50
_____	Sigmoidoscopy	Every 3–5 years for people over 50
_____	Tetanus/diphtheria vaccination	Every 10 years
_____	Influenza vaccination	Yearly for people over 65 or at special risk

For Men

_____	Testicular self-exam	Monthly

For Women

_____	Blood test for iron deficiency anemia	Pregnant women and high-risk infants
_____	Pap test	Every 3 years
_____	Breast self-exam	Monthly
_____	Mammography	Every 1–2 years for women 50–69 years

Note: The guidelines presented above represent the minimum tests recommended for people without symptoms. If you have symptoms or are at increased risk for certain conditions because of your medical or family history, additional tests may be advised. You should discuss your particular needs with your physician.

SOURCE: Adapted from 1996 U.S. Preventive Services Task Force Report.

WELLNESS WORKSHEET 79

Your Medicine Cabinet

Part I. What's Your Medicine Cabinet IQ?

Take this quiz to evaluate your knowledge of common medications; decide whether each statement is true (T) or false (F).

True   **False**

_____ _____   1. Acetaminophen (Tylenol) is safer for children than aspirin.

_____ _____   2. It's a good idea to keep some prescription antibiotics on hand in case you start to come down with a cold.

_____ _____   3. Hydrogen peroxide is a safe, effective antiseptic for cleaning cuts and scrapes.

_____ _____   4. Vitamin pills containing iron can be very toxic to children.

_____ _____   5. Taking vitamin C can help prevent you from catching a cold.

_____ _____   6. It's OK to share prescription medications with other people you know with the same physical complaints.

_____ _____   7. Calamine lotion is a good product for relieving minor itching.

_____ _____   8. Everyone should take vitamin supplements to boost his or her health.

Answers

1. True. Aspirin can cause a dangerous condition known as Reye's syndrome in children.
2. False. It is very dangerous to keep old antibiotics on hand. If you get a prescription for antibiotics, you should finish taking them even if you start to feel better.
3. True. Hydrogen peroxide is just as effective and less expensive than other OTC antiseptics.
4. True. Consuming iron-containing vitamins is the leading cause of poisoning in children under age 6. Be sure they are stored where children can't get them.
5. False. But some studies indicate that taking vitamin C may slightly diminish the severity of symptoms once a cold develops.
6. False. Taking someone else's prescription medicine can be very dangerous.
7. True. Calamine lotion can relieve itching from poison ivy or oak, insect bites, sunburn, and minor forms of dermatitis (skin irritations).
8. False. Most people who eat a healthy diet don't need vitamin supplements. There are some exceptions; ask your physician.

Scoring   Add up the number of questions you answered correctly.

7–8   Congratulations! You are very knowledgeable about self-care. Continue to educate yourself about home health issues.

4–6   You have some knowledge about self-care issues, but you need to be careful to read and follow all medication instructions.

0–3   Your lack of knowledge about self-care could put your health at risk. Read Chapter 21 carefully, and look for other ways to educate yourself about home health care issues.

(over)

Part II. Medicine Cabinet Check-up

Your home pharmacy should contain essential medical supplies. You can evaluate your pharmacy by completing the checklist below; consider purchasing any supplies that you do not check off.

Equipment

_____ Adhesive bandages

_____ Adhesive tape

_____ Cotton balls

_____ Elastic bandages

_____ Eye cup

_____ Gauze

_____ Heating pad or hot water bottle

_____ Ice pack

_____ Needle-nosed tweezers

_____ Sterile bandages

_____ Thermometer

Over-the-Counter Medications

_____ Antacids or acid reducers

_____ Antibacterial ointment or cream

_____ Antifungal preparations

_____ Antihistamines

_____ Aspirin, acetaminophen, ibuprofen, and/or naproxen sodium

_____ Burrow's solution

_____ Cough suppressant and expectorant

_____ Decongestant tablets or nose sprays

_____ Eye drops and artificial tears

_____ Hemorrhoid preparation

_____ Hydrocortisone cream

_____ Kaolin/pectate or loperamide

_____ Milk of magnesia or a bulk laxative

_____ Povidone iodine

_____ Sodium bicarbonate

_____ Sunscreen (SPF 15+)

_____ Syrup of ipecac

_____ Throat lozenges, spray, or gargle

Name _____ Section _____ Date _____

You can avoid communication problems with your physician by becoming fluent in some basic medical terminology. Begin by testing yourself on the following useful terms.

1. Adipose
   a. Fatty
   b. Additional X rays
   c. Totaling the bill

2. Ambulatory
   a. Transported by ambulance
   b. Able to walk
   c. Unable to walk

3. Analgesic
   a. Painkiller
   b. Rectal medicine
   c. Antibiotic

4. Antipyretic
   a. Bleeding gums
   b. Antacid
   c. Fever reducer

5. Atrophy
   a. Prize for best patient
   b. Weight loss
   c. Shrinkage of muscle or other tissue

6. Benign
   a. Noncancerous
   b. Fast-growing
   c. Cancerous

7. Congenital
   a. Friendly disposition
   b. A disorder of the genitals
   c. Condition present at birth

8. Contraindicated
   a. Recommended
   b. To be avoided
   c. Makes no difference

9. Dermatitis
   a. Tight skin
   b. Inflammation of the skin
   c. Numbness of the skin

10. Edema
    a. Swelling
    b. Pertaining to an enema
    c. Bruising

11. Etiology
    a. The study of eating
    b. The study of nutrition
    c. Pertaining to the causes of disease

12. Febrile
    a. High in fiber
    b. Feverish
    c. Weak

13. Hematoma
    a. Bruise
    b. Broken toe
    c. Iron deficiency

14. Hemorrhage
    a. Bleeding
    b. Pertaining to hemorrhoids
    c. Old blood

15. Idiopathic
    a. Of lower intelligence
    b. Not able to walk a straight line
    c. Of unknown cause

16. Lesion
    a. Any sore or wound
    b. A group of health practitioners
    c. Relief from stress

17. Negative test result
    a. The patient has a disorder
    b. The patient doesn't have the disorder
    c. The patient died

18. Parenteral
    a. Disease inherited from parents
    b. Medicine given by parents
    c. Medicine given by injection

(over)

19. Prognosis
    a. Disease of the nose
    b. A chronic condition
    c. Expected outcome of a disease

20. Pruritis
    a. Infection producing pus
    b. Itching
    c. Of highest purity

21. Psychogenic
    a. Of unsound mind
    b. Having an emotional origin
    c. Having a genetic origin

22. Q.I.D.
    a. Take four times a day
    b. Take for four days
    c. "Quit if disagreeable"

23. Sepsis
    a. Infection
    b. Cleanliness
    c. Waste removal

24. Sequela
    a. Aftereffect of a disease
    b. Quiet atmosphere
    c. Food poisoning

25. Subclinical
    a. The basement of the hospital
    b. A poorly equipped hospital
    c. Having no visible symptoms

26. Subcutaneous
    a. Not very pretty
    b. Beneath the skin
    c. Underfed

27. Syndrome
    a. Infected sinus
    b. A recurring infection
    c. A specific collection of symptoms

28. Systemic
    a. Affecting the whole body
    b. Methodical
    c. Cyst-forming

29. Topical
    a. Overheated
    b. On the surface
    c. Pertinent discussion

30. Urticaria
    a. Hives
    b. Burping
    c. Standing upright

Answers

1. a	2. b	3. a	4. c	5. c
6. a	7. c	8. b	9. b	10. a
11. c	12. b	13. a	14. a	15. c
16. a	17. b	18. c	19. c	20. b
21. b	22. a	23. a	24. a	25. c
26. b	27. c	28. a	29. b	30. a

Scoring

24–30   You're already well versed in medispeak, and because of that you rarely misunderstand your physician's explanations or instructions.

12–23   You're on your way to fluency, but you still need some assistance. That's why you often ask your physician to explain the words you are unfamiliar with, even though it sometimes makes you feel uncomfortable.

0–11   You need to invest in a medical dictionary for laypeople—and use it. Only then will you be able to change your feelings of intimidation to those of self-confidence.

SOURCE: Eileen Mazer, "Testing Your Knowledge of Medispeak." Copyright © 1997 Los Angles Times Syndicate. Reprinted by permission.

WELLNESS WORKSHEET 81

Getting the Most Out of Your Medical Care

To manage your own health successfully, you need to learn how to identify and manage medical problems and how to make the health care system work effectively for you. Review your knowledge of these areas by answering the questions below. Refer to your textbook if necessary.

1. List five things you should observe about symptoms.

   a. _____   d. _____

   b. _____   e. _____

   c. _____

2. What four general categories of symptoms require professional assistance?

   a. _____   c. _____

   b. _____   d. _____

3. List ten symptoms that indicate an urgent condition requiring a trip to the emergency room.

   a. _____   f. _____

   b. _____   g. _____

   c. _____   h. _____

   d. _____   i. _____

   e. _____   j. _____

4. List ten guidelines for using OTC medications safely and effectively.

   a. _____   f. _____

   b. _____   g. _____

   c. _____   h. _____

   d. _____   i. _____

   e. _____   j. _____

5. What can you do before an appointment with your physician that will help ensure good communication.

   _____

   List seven things you can do during an appointment that will help ensure good communication.

   a. _____

   b. _____

   c. _____

   d. _____

   (over)

e. _____

f. _____

g. _____

List three things you can do at the end of an appointment with your physician that will help ensure good communication.

a. _____

b. _____

c. _____

6. List five questions you should ask about a medical test recommended by your physician.

a. _____

b. _____

c. _____

d. _____

e. _____

7. What key questions should you ask when considering treatment options?

a. _____

b. _____

8. List seven important questions you should ask about a prescription medication.

a. _____

b. _____

c. _____

d. _____

e. _____

f. _____

g. _____

9. List four questions you should ask if your physician recommends surgery.

a. _____

b. _____

c. _____

d. _____

WELLNESS WORKSHEET 82

Selecting and Evaluating a Physician

Use the checklist below to evaluate your current physician or to choose a new one.

Yes   No

____ ____   The office appears to be run efficiently.

____ ____   The office atmosphere is friendly and reassuring.

____ ____   The receptionist is helpful when I call to make an appointment or arrive for a visit.

____ ____   Phone messages are passed on and phone calls returned in a timely manner.

____ ____   I am informed ahead of time if there will be any delays.

____ ____   The waiting area is rarely crowded.

____ ____   Privacy is provided when I am asked personal questions.

____ ____   The office accepts insurance, and requirements for payment are clearly explained.

____ ____   The physician seems thorough when taking my medical history.

____ ____   The physician gives me sufficient time and encouragement to completely describe my problem.

____ ____   The physician is receptive to my questions and concerns.

____ ____   The physician answers all my questions.

____ ____   The physician explains things clearly; he or she does not use so much medical jargon that I have difficulty understanding him or her.

____ ____   The physician explains the purpose and procedure for all medical tests.

____ ____   The physician clearly explains the diagnosis.

____ ____   The physician explains the reasons a particular drug is prescribed. He or she provides complete instructions for using the drug safely and effectively.

____ ____   Follow-up instructions are clearly given. I understand what my next step should be.

____ ____   The physician supports my decision to seek a second opinion when I feel it's necessary.

____ ____   The physician refers me to a specialist when indicated.

____ ____   The physician is willing to consult with me on the telephone when needed.

____ ____   Overall, the physician makes me feel comfortable with and confident of the services he or she is providing.

"No" answers indicate areas where your relationship with your physician or the running of the office may be less than ideal. Discuss any areas of concern with your physician. If things do not improve, consider changing physicians. Remember, your physician works for you.

(over)

INTERNET ACTIVITY

You can find information about many U.S. physicians from the online AMA Physician Select service, sponsored by the American Medical Association (http://www.ama-assn.org). This service lists the physician's address, area of specialty, training, and whether he or she is board certified; you can search for a physician by name or by location and area of specialty. Look up your current physician or one who is practicing at a clinic or a hospital near you. Or search for a particular type of specialist practicing in your area.

Physician's name: _____

Information obtained:

Name _____ Section _____ Date _____

WELLNESS WORKSHEET 83

Evaluating Health Insurance

The following questions are designed to help you evaluate different health insurance policies and choose the most appropriate one for you.

Costs

What is the yearly premium for the policy? _____

What is the deductible? _____

Is there a coinsurance system? If so, describe it. _____

_____

_____

Does the plan require a copayment for services? _____

If so, what is the system of copayments? _____

_____

Does the policy pay only the "usual" or "customary" fee for particular services? _____

Is there a maximum limit of coverage, either on a yearly basis or over the life of the policy? Are there limits

on the coverage of any particular conditions? _____

_____

(For point-of-service plans) If you visit a physician outside the plan, what percentage of the cost is covered?

_____

Coverage

What services does the policy cover? Check those that are covered; circle those you are most likely to need.

_____	Physician visits	_____	Preventive care
_____	Allergy testing and treatment	_____	Dental care
_____	Hospitalization	_____	Prenatal care and routine deliveries
_____	Prescription drugs	_____	Surgical costs, including anesthesia
_____	Second opinions	_____	X rays and lab services
_____	Ambulance service	_____	Emergency room care
_____	Mental health counseling/psychiatric care	_____	Substance abuse treatment
_____	Vision care	_____	Physical therapy
_____	Transfusions	_____	Out-of-town care
_____	Contraceptives	_____	Skilled nursing home care

(over)

Insel/Roth, *Core Concepts in Health*, Eighth Edition. © 1998 Mayfield Publishing Company. Chapter 22

List other services or supplies you may require and check whether or not these are covered under the policy.

Services/Supplies   **Covered?**

_____   _____

_____   _____

_____   _____

_____   _____

Restrictions/Exclusions

Are there exclusions for any preexisting conditions? If so, list any exclusions that would affect you. _____

_____

_____

_____

How long must you be free of symptoms before these conditions would be covered? _____

Is preauthorization required for any services? _____ Which services? _____

_____

Does the policy exclude particular conditions? If so, list any exclusions that may affect you. _____

_____

_____

Choice of Physician/Facilities

Are restrictions placed on your choice of physician? _____

_____

Would your current physician be covered by the plan? _____

Are there any restrictions on your choice of clinic, hospital, or emergency room? _____

_____

Waiting Period/Cancellation

Is the policy effective immediately? _____ If not, how long is the waiting period? _____

Is there a grace period for nonpayment of premiums or other fees? _____

Under what circumstances can the policy be cancelled? _____

_____

If you leave your job, can you maintain the policy by paying the premiums yourself? _____

Do you have any other options, such as temporarily extending the policy or changing to an individual policy?

_____

_____

WELLNESS WORKSHEET 84

Checklist for Preventing Unintentional Injuries

Put a check next to the answer that best describes your behavior, and fill in the requested information.

True **False**

Automobile/Truck Safety

_____ _____ I obey the speed limit at all times.

_____ _____ I follow the "three-second rule" to avoid following too closely: When the vehicle ahead passes a reference point, I count "one-thousand-one, one-thousand-two, one-thousand-three" (about 3 seconds). If I pass the reference point before I finish counting, I allow more space.

_____ _____ I slow down and allow more space between myself and the vehicle ahead when environmental conditions are not ideal (bad weather, poor road conditions, etc.).

_____ _____ I always wear a seatbelt, even when the vehicle has airbags.

_____ _____ I always securely strap infants or toddlers into appropriate child safety seats in the back seat of the car.

_____ _____ I never drink or use drugs and then drive.

_____ _____ I never get into a car if the driver has been drinking or using drugs.

_____ _____ I always signal when turning.

_____ _____ I always come to a complete stop at a stop sign or flashing red light.

_____ _____ I take special care at intersections: I look left, right, and then left again.

_____ _____ I don't pass on two-lane roads unless I'm in a designated passing area (broken line) or I have a clear view of oncoming traffic.

_____ _____ When given the choice between an interstate road and a rural road, I would choose to drive on the interstate.

_____ _____ When I buy a car, safety is one of my primary considerations.

_____ _____ I keep my car in good working order and regularly check:

_____ Tires _____ Brakes _____ Steering

_____ Lights _____ Windshield wipers _____ Oil and fluid levels

Motorcycle/Moped Safety

_____ _____ I always wear an approved helmet.

_____ _____ I always use eye protection (goggles, eye shields, or a windshield).

_____ _____ I wear long pants and a sturdy jacket to reduce injury in case of a fall.

_____ _____ I do everything possible to make myself more visible to other motorists.

_____ I wear light-colored clothing.

_____ I keep my headlight on at all times.

_____ I avoid changing lanes unless absolutely necessary.

_____ I avoid riding between lines of moving cars.

_____ _____ I have received proper training and adequate practice, and I have the skills to operate my motorcycle/moped safely.

(over)

Insel/Roth, *Core Concepts in Health,* Eighth Edition. © 1998 Mayfield Publishing Company. Chapter 23
Insel et al., *Core Concepts in Health,* Brief Eighth Edition. © 1998 Mayfield Publishing Company. Chapter 15

True   False

Cycling Safety

_____ _____ I know and follow the rules of the road.

_____ _____ I always ride with the flow of traffic.

_____ _____ I know and use proper hand signals.

_____ _____ I always ride defensively; I never assume that drivers have seen me.

_____ _____ I take special care in turning or crossing at corners and intersections.

_____ _____ I stop at all traffic lights and stop signs.

_____ _____ I keep my bike well-maintained.

_____ _____ I wear light-colored, reflective clothing that maximizes my visibility.

_____ _____ I always wear safety equipment:

_____ Helmet	_____ Gloves
_____ Appropriate footwear	_____ Reflective equipment at night
_____ Eye protection	_____ Pants clips or bands

_____ _____ I avoid busy roadways.

_____ _____ I use bike paths whenever possible.

Pedestrian Safety

_____ _____ I cross streets only in designated crosswalks.

_____ _____ I wait for a green light to cross the street.

_____ _____ I wear clothes that will make me more visible to drivers.

_____ _____ I never hitchhike.

Jogging Safety

_____ _____ I avoid busy roadways with poor visibility when possible.

_____ _____ I run against the flow of traffic.

_____ _____ I dress to be highly visible to drivers.

_____ _____ I jog during the day.

_____ _____ I don't listen to a radio or tape with headphones while jogging.

Swimming/Boating Safety

_____ _____ I do not attempt to swim distances that are beyond my physical capabilities.

_____ _____ I avoid swimming in dangerous or uncertain locations or situations.

_____ _____ I avoid swimming long in water that is colder than 70°F.

_____ _____ I do not use drugs or alcohol before I swim or while boating.

_____ _____ I always swim with at least one other person.

_____ _____ When boating, I wear an appropriate personal flotation device (PFD).

_____ _____ I know and follow safe boating rules.

_____ _____ I check water depth before diving.

True   False

Sports Safety

_____ _____ I participate only in those sports in which I have sufficient skill to play safely.

_____ _____ I recognize and guard against any hazards commonly associated with the sports I choose.

_____ _____ I include appropriate exercises for conditioning, warming up, and cooling down.

_____ _____ I use proper safety equipment and appropriate facilities (e.g., helmets, eye protection, knee and elbow pads, etc.).

_____ _____ I know how to recognize and avoid heat-related illness.

For the sport you most commonly participate in, list three common hazards and three pieces of needed safety equipment.

1. _____   1. _____

2. _____   2. _____

3. _____   3. _____

Hiking/Backpacking/Outdoor Activity Safety

_____ _____ I never hike or backpack alone.

_____ _____ I always tell someone where I am going and when I plan to return.

_____ _____ I always bring a map, compass, first aid kit, and emergency supplies.

_____ _____ I obtain weather information before any outdoor trip and dress appropriately.

_____ _____ I bring an adequate supply of fluids and limit strenuous activity during hot, humid weather.

_____ _____ I wear layers of warm clothing and covering for my head and hands when outdoors during cold weather.

_____ _____ I bring warm liquids and equipment for producing heat or starting fires if I will be outdoors for a prolonged period during cold weather.

Hunting/Fishing Safety

_____ _____ I take firearm safety and hunter safety courses regularly and follow all recommendations.

_____ _____ I keep firearms unloaded when they are not actively in use (including while hiking, crossing streams or ditches, or climbing over fences).

_____ _____ I am aware of others when casting or shooting.

_____ _____ I store equipment properly when it is not in use.

_____ _____ I store ammunition and firearms securely and separately.

Home Safety

_____ _____ Rugs and carpets are skid-proof.

_____ _____ Bathtubs have handrails and non-slip mats.

_____ _____ Floors are kept clear of conditions and objects that can cause slippage:

_____ Liquids   _____ Sand or gravel

_____ Heavy wax coating   _____ Small objects (e.g., toys)

_____ Electrical cords

True   False

_____ _____   Stairs are maintained in a safe condition:

        _____ Well-lighted   _____ With secure handrails or bannisters

        _____ Kept clear

_____ _____   Ladders are sturdy and in good repair.

_____ _____   Cigarettes are extinguished and disposed of in ashtrays.

_____ _____   No one in the household smokes while in bed.

_____ _____   Electrical appliances, furnaces, and kerosene heaters are regularly checked to ensure proper functioning.

_____ _____   Portable heaters are used only when carefully monitored and are kept away from flammable items.

_____ _____   The residence is equipped with carbon monoxide detectors.

_____ _____   Electrical outlets are used correctly, not overloaded.

_____ _____   All floors in the residence are equipped with fire or smoke detectors.

_____ _____   Two fire escape routes have been planned ahead of time for every room, and each resident knows what route he or she should take.

_____ _____   Fire-extinguishing instruments are handy and in good working condition.

_____ _____   Residents know how to avoid excessive smoke inhalation and what to do if their clothes catch fire:

(fill in) _____

_____

_____ _____   Medications are stored out of reach of children.

_____ _____   Cleaners, pesticides, and other dangerous and ingestible substances are stored correctly:

        _____ Out of reach of children   _____ In their original containers

_____ _____   Cleaners, pesticides, and other dangerous substances are used only in areas with proper ventilation.

_____ _____   Residents know how to recognize the signs of poisoning.

_____ _____   Residents know what to do in case of poisoning.

_____ _____   Residents know whom to call in case of poisoning.

_____ _____   Residents are trained in:

        _____ First Aid   _____ CPR   _____ Heimlich maneuver

IN CASE OF EMERGENCY, CALL _____

IN CASE OF POISONING, CALL (POISON CONTROL CENTER) _____

Your answers here can help you identify behaviors that you should change. Consider planning a behavior change program to alter one or more of your risky behaviors. You will probably have more success eliminating risks from your home if you can get all residents to participate in your behavior change program.

Name _____ Section _____ Date _____

WELLNESS WORKSHEET 85

Driving Like a Pro

Along with safe cars, safety belts, air bags, and sobriety, driving skills are an important element in motor vehicle safety. Learn to drive defensively, avoiding dangerous situations and reacting intelligently in a crisis. To find out how well you drive already, try this defensive-driving quiz. (Some questions have more than one correct answer.)

1. The safest way to brake is
   a. as fast as possible
   b. as far in advance as possible

2. In moderate town traffic, with another car at a safe distance in front of you, you're being tailgated. What do you do?
   a. Tap the brakes and start to slow down— gradually—keeping an eye on the rearview mirror.
   b. Increase your speed to the allowable limit.
   c. Try to pass the car in front of you.
   d. Pull over to the right.

3. You are traveling 30 mph on a dry road. Safe following distance is:
   a. 1 car length
   b. 2 car lengths
   c. 5 car lengths

4. Preparing to change lanes on a multilane highway, which of the following should you do?
   a. Check your rearview mirror.
   b. Check your side mirror.
   c. Take your eyes off the road momentarily and glance at the lane you're planing to move into.
   d. Turn on your directional signal.
   e. Be aware of what traffic in front of you is doing.

5. You've swerved to the right to avoid a collision on a two-way highway, and your right wheels drop off the pavement and are riding on the shoulder. To get back on the road, you
   a. accelerate, cutting the wheel to the left.
   b. don't brake but take your foot off the accelerator. Hold the wheel steady. When the car slows, check the traffic and steer back onto the pavement.
   c. brake sharply and try to pull off the road altogether. When you've got the car under control, pull onto the road again.

6. On a two-way highway, in what's clearly marked as a no-pass zone with limited visibility, a car pulls out to pass you. Your best move is to
   a. speed up, hoping the car will move back behind you.
   b. ignore the car—it's not your problem.
   c. reduce your speed so the car can get around you faster.

7. The most important factor in defensive driving is
   a. quick reflexes
   b. anticipating trouble
   c. skill at vehicle handling
   d. strict observation of the law

8. Which of the following road conditions up ahead should tell you to reduce your speed?
   a. a deep pothole
   b. leaves on the pavement
   c. any bridge when the temperature is just above freezing

9. Your rear-wheel-drive car is skidding (see diagram). What's the safest reaction?

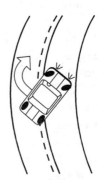

   a. Turn the wheel to the right.
   b. Turn the wheel to the left.
   c. Brake as hard as possible and avoid turning the wheel until you've stopped the car.

(over)

Insel/Roth, *Core Concepts in Health,* Eighth Edition. © 1998 Mayfield Publishing Company. Chapter 23
Insel et al., *Core Concepts in Health,* Brief Eighth Edition. © 1998 Mayfield Publishing Company. Chapter 15

10. In two-way highway traffic, an oncoming car suddenly pulls into your lane. What action do you take?

   a. Brake hard and sound your horn.
   b. Move quickly into the left lane.
   c. Blow your horn and head to the shoulder.

11. The best position for your hands on the steering wheel is
   a. at the 10:00 and 2:00 o'clock positions
   b. at the 8:00 and 4:00 o'clock positions
   c. wherever you're most comfortable
   d. at the 9:00 and 3:00 o'clock positions

12. True or false. Underinflated tires are safer, particularly in hot weather.

Answers

1. (b) A basic principle of defensive driving is never to get into a situation that calls for slamming on the brakes. This can throw you into a skid and injure you and your passengers.

2. (a) and (d), depending on circumstances. If the tailgater is daydreaming, tapping your brakes (and activating the brake lights) should wake him or her up. If the driver is being aggressive, you've politely given a signal to let up. If the tailgating doesn't stop, pull over as soon as you can and let the other car pass.

3. (c) On a dry road, going 30 mph, give yourself two to three seconds to stop, or about 5 car lengths. If you are driving faster, if the road is wet, if visibility is poor, or if you are tired, drop back more. To determine how close you are following, notice when the rear of the vehicle ahead passes a tree or other fixed point. Then count "one thousand one, one thousand two," and so on until you pass the same fixed point.

4. (all) All steps are essential, but some people forget (c). You always have a blind spot (about a car length behind you on either side) and may not be able to see an overtaking vehicle in either mirror. Always glance over your shoulder before making your move. The signal light turned on several seconds in advance will help protect you as well.

5. (b) Braking hard or jerking the wheel can cause you to skid into oncoming traffic. Don't brake but do reduce your speed and stay on a steady course. Then, after checking traffic, make a sharp quarter turn to the left to put yourself back on the road and then straighten out.

6. (c) Passing is always a cooperative venture. If this reckless driver has a head-on collision, you might be hurt, too.

7. (b) Obeying the law and vehicle-handling skills are all important. But anticipating trouble up ahead and acting to prevent it can make the speed of your reflexes far less important and thus may prevent many collisions.

8. (all) The pothole may only jar you, but it could damage your car or even cause you to lose control. Leaves can send you into a skid. And even though there's no ice on the road, a bridge is about 6°F colder than a highway and may be hazardous when the road is not.

9. (b) Turn the wheel straight down your lane. That is, if your rear wheels are skidding left, as in the diagram, turn with the skid—that is, to the left. Don't brake; it increases skidding.

10. (c) Don't move left, which could put you in someone else's pathway. Always move right when heading off the road.

11. (d) And some expert drivers recommend that you hook your thumbs lightly over the horizontal spokes. This gives you a feel for the front tires and is a good way to get a quick grip if you strike a pothole.

12. False. An underinflated tire is more likely to skid, whether in hot weather or on wet or icy pavement. Because underinflation allows a tire to "flap" slightly and thus to create more heat, it's also more likely to blow out. Even for desert driving, keep tires at the recommended maximum air pressure and check them weekly. The number should be printed on the side of the tires; or check the instruction manual if the car still has its original tires.

SOURCE: Adapted from Driving through the 90s. 1994. *University of California at Berkeley Wellness Letter,* July. Driving like the pros. 1989. *University of California at Berkeley Wellness Letter*, October. Reprinted by permission from the University of California Berkeley Wellness Letter. Copyright © 1989, 1994 Health Letter Associates.

Name _____ Section _____ Date _____

WELLNESS WORKSHEET 86

Personal Safety Checklist

Are you doing all you can to protect yourself from violence and injuries? The following list of statements relate to intentional injury incidents that can occur in a variety of settings. Put a check next to those statements that are true for you and fill in the requested information.

At Home

_____ My home has good lighting.

_____ Doors are secured with effective locks (deadbolts).

_____ All unused doors and windows are securely locked.

_____ I always lock all windows and doors when I go out.

_____ I have a dog and/or post "Beware of Dog" signs.

_____ Landscaping around the home doesn't provide opportunities for concealment.

_____ Keys are hidden in a secure, non-obvious place.

_____ I do not give anyone the opportunity to duplicate my keys.

_____ The front door has a peephole.

_____ I do not open my door to strangers or allow them into my home or yard.

_____ I ask to see ID or call to verify that repair and utility workers are legitimate.

_____ I use my initials in phone directory listings.

_____ My answering machine message does not imply that I live alone or am not home.

_____ Everyone in the household knows how to call for help.

_____ My neighbors and I have a system for alerting one another in case of an emergency.

_____ I participate in a neighborhood watch program.

On the Street

_____ I avoid walking alone, especially at night or in less-populous areas.

_____ I dress in clothing that allows freedom of movement.

_____ I walk purposefully, in an alert and confident manner.

_____ I walk on the outside of the sidewalk, facing traffic.

_____ I check routes to my destination before leaving so as not to appear lost.

_____ I never hitchhike.

_____ I carry valuables in a secure or concealed location.

_____ I have my keys ready when I approach my vehicle or home.

_____ I carry change for a telephone call, fare for public transportation, and a whistle to blow if I am attacked or harassed.

_____ I keep alert for suspicious behavior, and I keep at least two arm lengths between myself and strangers.

_____ I know what to do if I feel threatened or if someone grabs me: _____

(over)

Insel/Roth, *Core Concepts in Health,* Eighth Edition. © 1998 Mayfield Publishing Company. Chapter 23
Insel et al., *Core Concepts in Health,* Brief Eighth Edition. © 1998 Mayfield Publishing Company. Chapter 15

In My Car

_____ My car is in good working condition.

_____ I carry emergency supplies in my car.

_____ I keep my gas tank at least half full.

_____ When driving, I keep doors locked and windows rolled up at least three-quarters of the way.

_____ I park my car in well-lighted areas or parking garages.

_____ I lock my car when I leave it.

_____ I check the interior of my car before unlocking it and getting in.

_____ I don't pick up strangers. If I see a vehicle in distress: _____

_____

_____ I note the location of emergency call boxes, or I have a cellular phone in my car.

_____ I use caution if my car breaks down: _____

_____

_____ When I stop at a light or stop sign, I stop far enough behind the car in front to allow room to maneuver in case of emergency.

_____ I use caution if I am involved in a minor crash or bumped intentionally: _____

_____

_____ I do not get into arguments with drivers of other vehicles.

On Public Transportation

_____ I wait in populated, well-lighted areas.

_____ I sit near the driver or conductor.

_____ I sit in a single seat or an outside seat.

_____ I check routes and times in advance, and confirm before boarding that the bus, subway, or train is bound for my destination.

On Campus

_____ Door and window locks are secure.

_____ Halls and stairwells have adequate lighting.

_____ I do not give dorm or residence keys to others.

_____ I keep my door locked.

_____ I do not allow strangers into my room.

_____ I do not walk, jog, or exercise alone at night.

_____ I use campus escort services or walk with friends.

_____ I know the areas that security guards patrol and stay where they can see or hear me if possible.

Your answers here can help you identify behaviors that you should change. Consider planning a behavior change strategy to alter one or more of your risky behaviors.

WELLNESS WORKSHEET 87

Violence in Relationships

Part I. Recognizing the Potential for Abusiveness

If you are concerned that a man you are involved with has the potential for violence, observe his behavior and ask yourself these questions.

1. What is this person's attitude toward women? How does he treat his mother and his sister? How does he work with female students, female colleagues, or a female boss? How does he treat your women friends?

2. What is his attitude toward your autonomy? Does he respect the work you do and the way you do it? Or does he put it down, or tell you how to do it better, or encourage you to give it up? Does he tell you he'll take care of you?

3. How self-centered is he? Does he want to spend leisure time on your interests or his? Does he listen to you? Does he remember what you say?

4. Is he possessive or jealous? Doe he want to spend every minute with you? Does he cross-examine you about things you do when you're not with him?

5. What happens when things don't go the way he wants them to? Does he blow up? Does he always have to get his way?

6. Is he moody, mocking, critical, or bossy? Do you feel as if you're "walking on eggshells" when you're with him?

7. Do you feel you have to avoid arguing with him?

8. Does he drink too much or use drugs?

9. Does he refuse to use condoms or take other precautions for safer sex?

(over)

Insel/Roth, *Core Concepts in Health,* Eighth Edition. © 1998 Mayfield Publishing Company. Chapter 23
Insel et al., *Core Concepts in Health,* Brief Eighth Edition. © 1998 Mayfield Publishing Company. Chapter 15

Experts summarize their advice to women this way: Listen to your own uneasiness, and stay from any man who disrespects women, who wants or needs you intensely and exclusively, and who has a knack for getting his own way almost all the time.

Part II. Recognizing Signs of Abuse

Yes   No

_____ _____ 1. Does your partner constantly criticize you, blame you for things that are not your fault, or verbally degrade you?

_____ _____ 2. Does he humiliate you in front of others?

_____ _____ 3. Is he suspicious or jealous? Does he accuse you of being unfaithful or monitor your mail or phone calls?

_____ _____ 4. Does he "track" all your time? Does he discourage you from seeing friends and family?

_____ _____ 5. Does he prevent you from getting or keeping a job or attending school? Does he control your shared resources or restrict your access to money?

_____ _____ 6. Has he ever pushed, slapped, hit, kicked, bitten, or restrained you? Thrown an object at you? Used a weapon on you?

_____ _____ 7. Has he ever destroyed or damaged your personal property or sentimental items?

_____ _____ 8. Has he ever forced you to have sex or to do something sexually you didn't want to do?

_____ _____ 9. Does he anger easily when drinking or taking drugs?

_____ _____ 10. Has he ever threatened to harm you or your children, friends, pets, or property?

_____ _____ 11. Has he ever threatened to blackmail you if you leave?

If you answered yes to one or more of these questions, you may be experiencing domestic abuse. If you believe you or your children are in imminent danger, look in your local telephone directory for a women's shelter, or call 911. If you want information, referrals to a program in your area, or assistance, contact one of the organizations listed in For More Information in Chapter 23 of your textbook (Chapter 15 in the brief version).

INTERNET ACTIVITY

Research Web resources relating to date rape or domestic violence; use the Web sites listed in your text and/or do a Web search. What resources are available for victims and abusers? Are referrals to support groups or legal help provided? Are there suggestions for friends of victims or concerned citizens and communities? Write a brief description of the most helpful site you locate.

Topic: _____

Site visited (URL): _____

Description:

SOURCES: Family Violence Prevention Fund. 1996. *Take Action Against Domestic Violence.* San Francisco, Calif.: Family Violence Prevention Fund. How to tell if you're in an abusive situation. 1994. *San Francisco Chronicle,* 24 June. Jones, A. 1994. *Next Time She'll Be Dead.* Boston: Beacon Press.

WELLNESS WORKSHEET 88

Facts About Environmental Health

Review your knowledge of important issues in environmental health by answering the questions below. Refer to your textbook if necessary.

1. List two current problems regarding clean water and a possible solution for each.

   a. _____

   _____

   b. _____

   _____

2. What are the major components of household trash? What are some of the problems with trash disposal?

   _____

   _____

   _____

   _____

3. List three factors that contribute to population growth and three factors that may limit it.

   a. _____   a. _____

   b. _____   b. _____

   c. _____   c. _____

4. What is a temperature inversion, and why is it dangerous?

   _____

   _____

   _____

   _____

5. What is the greenhouse effect?

   _____

   _____

   _____

   _____

(over)

Insel/Roth, *Core Concepts in Health*, Eighth Edition. © 1998 Mayfield Publishing Company. Chapter 24
Insel et al., *Core Concepts in Health*, Brief Eighth Edition. © 1998 Mayfield Publishing Company. Chapter 16

6. What is the ozone layer, and why is it important to human health?

_____

_____

_____

How and where does thinning of the ozone layer occur?

_____

_____

_____

7. What is acid precipitation, and how does it occur?

_____

_____

_____

8. List and describe two current chemical pollution problems. What are the effects of each chemical? How do people come in contact with them?

a. _____

_____

b. _____

_____

9. What negative effects can occur when an individual is exposed to loud and persistent noise?

_____

_____

List three strategies for avoiding excess noise.

a. _____

b. _____

c. _____

10. What is biodiversity, and why is it important?

_____

_____

_____

Name _____ Section _____ Date _____

WELLNESS WORKSHEET 89

Environmental Health Checklist: Lessening Your Impact on the Environment

The following statements relate to your impact on the environment. Put a check next to any statement that is true for you.

_____ I ride my bike, walk, use public transportation, or carpool in a fuel-efficient vehicle whenever possible.

_____ I keep my car tuned up and well-maintained.

_____ I use only unleaded gas.

_____ My car tires are inflated at the proper pressure.

_____ I avoid quick starts and drive within the speed limit.

_____ I don't use my car's air conditioner when opening the window would suffice.

_____ I keep my car's air conditioner in good working order and have it serviced at a station that recycles, rather than releases, CFCs.

_____ My residence is well-insulated.

_____ I have an energy-efficient refrigerator, which I keep in good working order.

_____ Where possible, I use compact fluorescent bulbs instead of incandescent bulbs.

_____ I turn off lights and appliances when they are not in use.

_____ I avoid turning on heaters and air conditioners.

_____ The sinks in my residence have aerators installed in them.

_____ The showers in my residence have low-flow showerheads.

_____ I have a water-saving toilet, or I have a water displacement device.

_____ I fix any faucets that leak.

_____ I run the washing machine, dryer, and dishwasher only when they have full loads.

_____ I use a china mug and metal spoon for coffee and tea rather than disposable cups and stirrers.

_____ I recycle newspapers, glass, cans, paper, and other materials.

_____ I have a compost pile or bin for my organic garbage, or I take my organic garbage to a community composting center.

_____ I don't pour toxic materials (bleach, motor oil, etc.) down the sink.

_____ If I am unsure of the proper way to dispose of something, I contact my local health department or environmental health office.

_____ I take showers instead of baths.

_____ I don't run water while brushing my teeth, shaving, or washing dishes.

_____ I dry my hair with a towel rather than a hair dryer.

_____ I take my own bag along when I go shopping.

(over)

Insel/Roth, *Core Concepts in Health,* Eighth Edition. © 1998 Mayfield Publishing Company. Chapter 24
Insel et al., *Core Concepts in Health,* Brief Eighth Edition. © 1998 Mayfield Publishing Company. Chapter 16

_____ When shopping, I choose products with the least amount of packaging.

_____ I buy products in bulk.

_____ I choose recycled and recyclable products.

_____ I choose the least toxic products available.

_____ I buy organic produce or produce that is in season and has been grown locally.

_____ I store food in glass jars and reusable plastic containers rather than using plastic wrap.

_____ Whenever possible, I use long-lasting or reusable products (refillable pens and rechargeable batteries, for example).

_____ I avoid products containing methyl chloroform (1, 1, 1-trichloroethane) and halon.

_____ I snip or rip plastic six-pack rings before discarding them. (When birds or animals get them stuck on their necks or bills, they can strangle or starve to death.)

_____ I don't buy products made from endangered species.

_____ When hiking or camping, I never leave anything behind.

Statements that you have not checked can help you identify behaviors that you can change to improve environmental health. To change some of the behaviors listed, you may need the cooperation of your family and/or roommate(s). If there are environmental issues that are important to you, you can go beyond individual action by informing others, joining and volunteering your time to organizations working on environmental problems, and contacting your elected representatives.

INTERNET ACTIVITY

Writing letters to elected officials is one way you can become more involved in promoting environmental health. Choose one of your representatives—local, state, or United States Congress—and locate her or his e-mail address. The Library of Congress has a Web page with links to many directories for members of Congress (http://lcweb.loc.gov/global/legislative/email.html). Other officials can be located through Web searches (enter a name into a search engine). Fill in the e-mail address of your representative, and briefly describe how you located it.

Name: _____

Position: _____

E-mail address: _____

How located:

Name _____ Section _____ Date _____

WELLNESS WORKSHEET 90

Recycling and Shopping Planner

Part I. Recyclables Reminder

Research the recycling facilities in your area. For each type of recyclable, fill in where it can be recycled and what preparation is required (for example, removing labels or tying bundles).

ALUMINUM AND STEEL CANS

	Type	*Can be recycled at (location):*
____	Aluminum cans	_____
____	Foil OK?	
____	Pie plates, frozen food trays, etc. OK?	
____	Steel cans	_____

Preparation: _____

_____

_____

GLASS

	Type	*Can be recycled at (location):*
____	Clear glass	_____
____	Green glass	_____
____	Amber glass	_____

Preparation: _____

_____

_____

PAPER

	Type	*Can be recycled at (location):*
____	Newspaper	_____
____	Corrugated cardboard	_____
____	Brown paper bags OK?	
____	Office paper	_____
____	Laser-printed paper OK?	
____	Mixed papers	_____
____	Acceptable papers are:	_____
____	Glossy paper	_____
____	Glued bindings OK?	

Preparation: _____

_____

_____

(over)

PLASTIC

	Type	*Can be recycled at (location):*
_____	1 PET or PETE	_____
_____	2 HDPE	_____
_____	6 PS	_____
_____	Others?	_____

Preparation: _____

_____

_____

OTHER

	Type	*Can be recycled at (location):*
_____	Batteries (home)	_____
_____	Batteries (car)	_____
_____	Motor oil	_____
_____	Paint	_____
_____		_____
_____		_____

Preparation: _____

_____

_____

Part II. Critical Shopping for Environmental Health

You can promote environmental health by purchasing sustainable products whenever possible. A product is sustainable if it is made, used, and disposed of in such a way that it could continue to be made, used, and disposed of again and again. To begin building your environmental shopping skills, choose a product and ask yourself the following questions about it.

Product: _____

1. Do I really need this product? Why? (Every product you *don't* buy saves resources and eliminates waste.)

2. Is the product safe to use? (Choose nontoxic alternatives whenever possible.)

3. Is the product practical, durable, well made, of good quality, with a timeless design? Will I be able to keep it for a long time before replacing it? (Products that last are better for the environment.)

4. Is the product made from renewable or recycled materials?

5. How will I dispose of the product, and what environmental impact will that disposal have?

6. What kind of package does the product have?

7. How far has the product been shipped to reach the retail outlet? (Products produced locally for use fewer resources and produce less pollution during transport.)

8. Is the product a good value for the money? Is the environmental health benefit the product provides worth the extra cost?

SOURCE: Adapted from Dadd-Redalia, D. 1994. *Sustaining the Earth.* New York: Hearst Books. Copyright © 1994 Debra Dadd-Redalia. By permission of Hearst Books, an imprint of William Morrow Company, Inc.